D1616385

More Advance Praise for *Sleep to Heal*

"There are many actions you can take that make you a successful entrepreneur, and getting enough sleep is one of them. Until I read *Sleep to Heal*, that advice would have fallen into the 'do as I say, not as I do' category. But this book has already positively impacted my life, making me more aware and alert and revitalizing my business by awakening my brain. I'm certain it can do the same for you and your small business!"

—Rieva Lesonsky, bestselling author and founder
GrowBiz Media and SmallBusinessCurrents.com

"Sleep is where it all starts and ends. I have learned so much about my own health and have taken his advice to heart. The impact of technology was a big one for me, and learning about how my body heals with sleep has been life-changing for my family. So many struggle with something we can all get for free. Dr. Singh and his knowledge can change the world."

—Angela Ganote, news anchor for Fox59 Morning
News, Indiana's #1 rated show

"Dr. Singh sheds light on topics that have material impact on reducing errors in fields like medicine and aviation. Optimizing sleep may very well be the magic pill we have been searching for to heal our collective ails!"

—S. R. Srinivasan, MD, ICU physician, and certified flight instructor

SLEEP TO HEAL

SLEEP TO HEAL

7 Simple Steps to Better Sleep

ABHINAV SINGH, MD, MPH, FAASM

with Charlotte Jensen

Charlotte Jensen

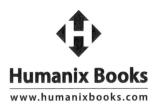

Humanix Books

www.humanixbooks.com

Humanix Books

SLEEP TO HEAL

Humanix Books, P.O. Box 20989, West Palm Beach, FL 33416, USA
www.humanixbooks.com | info@humanixbooks.com

Humanix Books is a division of Humanix Publishing, LLC. Its trademark, consisting of the words "Humanix Books," is registered in the Patent and Trademark Office and in other countries.

Disclaimer: The information presented in this book is not specific medical advice for any individual and should not substitute medical advice from a health professional. If you have (or think you may have) a medical problem, speak to your doctor or a health professional immediately about your risk and possible treatments. Do not engage in any care or treatment without consulting a medical professional.

ISBN: 9-781-63006-234-7 (Hardcover)
ISBN: 9-781-63006-235-4 (E-book)

Printed in the United States of America
10 9 8 7 6 5 4 3 2 1

To Vidhya, the queen of my universe,
and Zoe, our warrior princess
—**ABHINAV SINGH, MD**

For Rhys, who brightens every day
—**CHARLOTTE JENSEN**

Contents

Part III:
What Does Better Sleep Look Like?

Foreword

During my tenure as CEO of Indiana Internal Medicine Consultants from 1997 to 2016, I hired close to 70 MDs and NPs. I made a lot of good hires, a few bad ones, and several exceptional ones. Abhinav Singh was clearly one of the latter. Soon, as you read this book, you will undoubtedly understand why.

Too many MDs approach their workday as if they are punching a time clock—it's just a job, a necessary burden. But some do indeed demonstrate a true passion for their vocation. They understand that the opportunity to practice medicine is a privilege despite burdensome electronic medical records or the pressures that accumulate when staffing is short or when partners are out with COVID.

Some physicians are able to compartmentalize the frustrations that we face, deal with them as need be, yet still have the capacity to be excited by the intellectual challenges of our work and fulfilled by the opportunity to help another during their time of need. For one with true empathy, the effort it takes to make the additional call after hours to a concerned family member or search for a journal article late at night to assist in the management of a complex problem is not burdensome but rather the natural manifestation of the compassion modeled by the best in our profession. Dr. Singh is an exceptional clinician embodying all these attributes and brings positive energy and passion that jump off the pages that follow.

Interestingly, prior to reading this book, I spent some time reflecting on my own nearly 40-year career as an internist—one that encompassed primary care, office consultative practice, hospital-based internal medicine, critical care, and end-of-life palliative care. I loved my office years providing primary care, though eventually acute care responsibilities at the hospital plus administrative duties took me away from office practice. Yet as I thought about primary care and preventive medicine, my first thoughts landed on the holy trinity of health maintenance easily accessible to all: nutrition, exercise, and quality sleep. Like Dr. Singh, I pondered the challenges potentially imposed by the first two in contrast to the third, which requires no sacrifice but rather just discipline, which I believe to be readily attainable if one is properly educated and motivated.

This is the clinician's challenge. Establishment of trust and confidence is essential as we try to lead our patients to optimal health. While many clinicians may be book smart, not all are able to convey their message in a manner that promotes healing. Not all are relatable; you wouldn't want to sit down and enjoy a nice cold beer with many. By the time you finish reading this book, however, you will know that you have a new friend, and you will want to join Dr. Singh in a jam session or sit with him and watch as his face lights up talking about his wife or daughter. And you will be awestruck by his knowledge of and passion for sleep medicine as he makes his case for optimizing the third of his "three pillars" of good health: exercise, nutrition, and sleep.

This book is wonderfully written. It is a public health primer on the healing nature of quality sleep that reads as part history, part coming-of-(professional)-age story, part peer-reviewed medical literature, and part real-life medical vignettes, all skillfully woven together with folksy anecdotes and relatable analogies such that the reader cannot help but be richly entertained while still being educated—not just medically but also from a broader philosophy-of-life perspective. Dr. Singh is an optimist, an idealist, and he is in *your* corner, *our* corners. He is determined to make this world a better place; determined to invite all of us to be open to new possibilities; determined to start a sleep revolution. I, for one, am not betting against him!

As shared by Dr. Singh, one of our basic tenets of medical practice is first to "do no harm." Oftentimes, we just need to get out of the way and let time show us the path to healing. Pills are not always the answer. I personally am loath to prescribe medicine unless absolutely necessary (as my children and wife will attest!). Evolution reflects unlimited and unrestricted time and experimentation and has identified powerful healers. Across multiple species, Dr. Singh explains, the adaptive evolution of sleep physiology attests to its healing properties. All would be wise—and will live longer and better—to heed sage medical advice springing from lessons of nature still being discovered. *Sleep to Heal* makes the compelling case for each of us to utilize the simple tools at our disposal to take full advantage of what nature tries to teach us.

BILL BUFFIE, MD
Indianapolis, Indiana

Introduction

When people think of a sleep physician, the image that comes to mind isn't of someone who steps through crowded city streets, knocking on strangers' doors. But in some kind of wonderful and destined way, that's exactly how I started out on this fascinating journey—and ultimately what led me to where I am today, as one of only around 2,000 sleep specialists in the United States granted fellowship in the American Academy of Sleep Medicine.

Back in the late 1990s, not long after Bombay became officially known as Mumbai, I was a young medical student with no direction yet in which field to specialize. Surgery? No, that didn't interest me. Cardiac? Not my thing. All my peers at Topiwala National Medical College, Nair Hospital, were fascinated by complex diseases and anatomy, but me, not as much. My draw to medicine came from somewhere else: For one thing, I could be the first doctor in my family. That was appealing. But even deeper than that, this idea of *health* tugged at me more than *disease*. Public health—not just here in Mumbai, or even India, but globally. I wanted to find a way to bring health to the world.

This realization didn't begin to take shape until, as part of my training, I worked to help vaccinate the city's population against polio. In India, preventive medicine finally makes its way into the medical school curriculum in a student's final year, and for me, that coincided with a huge campaign to achieve mass immunity. Polio was eradicated in the United States in 1979, but when I was still a student in India, this important milestone had yet to be reached. In fact, it didn't even happen until years later, in 2014.

And so in 2001, I found myself with a few other medical students winding my way through narrow alleyways and streets, stepping over garbage, and knocking on doors in the poorest neighborhoods of Mumbai. My hope was that the concerned mothers who opened those doors, clutching their babies and with curious faces peeking out from behind their saris, would give me a chance and hear what I had to say. They all conveyed the same worries: "Why should I let you do this? What is this?" It was not lost on me how immensely important this job was and that I must calm their fears. Not just so that I could squeeze some life-giving drops into hundreds of little mouths but because if I could explain polio vaccination to every mother effectively, in a way she could understand, she would then tell her family, and then they would tell their families, and so on.

One patient at a time is not an efficient way of improving public health. But what if there could be a domino effect, with this one tiny spark of awareness spreading exponentially? I got really excited thinking about this idea of eradicating polio and making the whole society healthy! I call this 360 degrees of awareness, a philosophy I'm passionate about and that you will learn more about in this book.

Awakening to Sleep

By the time I made my way to the United States in the fall of 2002 to get my master's in public health at the University of Illinois at Chicago, sleep medicine as a specialty still hadn't crossed my mind. I had no idea the subject could be so fascinating. Medical schools hardly even touch it—we had just two lectures on sleep, and the second one I ducked out of because it was the "easy, boring one" that everyone just skipped. (Yes, I am laughing at my young self right now.)

I also didn't know until I arrived on campus that in just a couple of weeks after stepping off the plane at O'Hare, my first bill for $16,000 in tuition would be due. What?! My medical school in India had been basically free! I had taken out a loan to buy my plane ticket, and here I was running dangerously low on the remainder.

My sister, who worked in tech locally, advised me to look for a research assistant position that might help me pay some bills and maybe even some tuition. I scrambled and printed 80 resumes and slid them under various faculty office doors. (Job hunting was still done the old-fashioned way at this time.) A few places called; most didn't. I desperately needed something, but nothing panned out.

Until the sleep lab at the Center for Narcolepsy, Sleep, and Health Research called me back.

And so, with three days left to find a way to earn some money, I found myself sitting across from a prominent researcher who asked me point-blank, "What do you know about sleep?"

I paused for a few seconds, knowing I had to ace this answer. I had a $110,000 degree to pay for. On the wall behind her was some framed artwork depicting the human brain, and as I stared at it, I realized that my brain knew very little about sleep. But surely I couldn't tell her that! If only I had attended that sleep lecture back in medical school.

I said, "Not much . . . but I know we all need it." I couldn't give the answer she was looking for, but it was the truth. The confidence I conveyed hid my feelings inside, and I envisioned my chances for a scholarship and my dream life in America slowly slipping away.

She smiled and said, "Using your medical background, would you be interested in helping us recruit patients with sleep disorders?"

"Yes!"

"Great! We will be able to take care of your grad school fees this semester."

I thought, *Wait a second: What exactly does "take care of" mean?* Stunned and filled with joy, I had no words. My mind scrambled, trying to convert dollars into rupees: 16,000 × 50 is . . . how much exactly?

Concerned I had said nothing and thinking it might not be enough for me, she added, "How about we add a stipend of $800 a month for 20 hours a week?"

Coming back to my senses, I realized I had just hit a giant jackpot. "Wow! That is so kind!" I said. We shook hands, and she asked me to show up at the sleep research center later that week for orientation.

And so began my first baby steps into this enchanting universe of sleep. I learned a ton and spent long hours reviewing polysomnograms (sleep studies that gather data from your brain and body during sleep) and patient sleep questionnaires and interviewing thousands of patients with sleep disorders for the center's research. My work there meant my entire tuition for the next three years would be paid for in full—except that I almost blew the whole thing a few months later . . . when I *fell asleep on the job* in front of my boss and the patient in the sleep lab because I was so sleep deprived. (In my defense, the 20-minute sleep study was happening in a dark room while I had to relax in a recliner. But still!)

Here's the thing about sleep: Just as I answered in my interview, we do all need it. Each and every one of us. As you will see throughout this book, but especially in chapter 2, depriving your body and mind of sleep can mean any number of negative consequences—including falling asleep at the exact wrong time.

As for me, I walked out of the lab that day with the heaviest heart. Here I was, finally living my dream. I'd stepped inside my own real-life version of *Chicago Hope*, my favorite TV show when I lived in India. And now my sleep deprivation was on the verge of depriving me of my biggest dream. I probably would have lost everything had I zonked out while working in any other specialty: Neurology. Anesthesiology. Emergency room medicine. You name it.

But I didn't. My boss at the time was very understanding. He tapped me on the shoulder to wake me and suggested I should probably go to my next class so I wouldn't be late. He knew I was this young, busy medical student exhausted by the university–sleep lab–study–library cycle. But that's when I realized for myself that something had to change. I could never make that mistake again. I had also begun to understand firsthand, in my work from interviewing our sleep subjects, how sleep disorders could really capsize people's lives. But I also saw how the right treatments led to incredible transformations. And so I took protecting my sleep seriously and to heart from that point on. Something I hope you, too, take away from this book.

I knew sleep was my calling when I got the golden opportunity to join one of the nation's finest sleep medicine fellowship training programs at Northwestern University under the direction of my mentor, Phyllis Zee, MD, PhD. An internationally recognized researcher, Dr. Zee is a prominent thought leader in the field of sleep medicine and a physician with a passion for teaching. My final year of training convinced me: This is it! Sleep medicine is my dream career!

13.5 Million Minutes

As we continue to make exciting discoveries in the field of sleep science, I see an awakening dawning for all of us as the idea that better sleep equals a more fulfilling life becomes more widespread. You don't need to be suffering from a sleep disorder to benefit from this book—although if you are, you will. All of us can revitalize our health and happiness simply by optimizing the quality and quantity of our sleep. Optimal sleep is like installing guardrails *before* a disorder has a chance to creep in. It's your head-to-toe invisible armor that always works to protect you from ill health. Sleep will not just prevent a multitude of ailments, both mental and physical, but also assist in healing, and in ways we don't fully understand. It's so magnificent to think about how every cell of your body gets a "car wash and detail" while you sleep. (More about this in chapter 4.) And that's just the beginning.

In my speeches, I like to talk about this idea of sleep as a mutual fund, where the goal is to deposit 13.5 million minutes ($13.5 million) over the years of your life and reap health dividends. That number, 13.5 million, is the magic number of minutes we should all hopefully sleep in an average lifetime of around 80 years.

You can think of it another way too: What if sleep was like a hotel you check into every night? You can check into the $500-per-night five-star hotel (500 minutes = 8.3 hours) or the $250-per-night two-star motel (250 minutes = 4.1 hours). Which hotel would you rather sleep in? If you're like most of us, the $500-per-night hotel looks more comfortable. It's the fancier one with a better bed, fluffier pillows, and softer sheets, in the prime part of town. It's the one that ensures a beautiful night's rest. Although $500 adds up to a little more than eight hours per night of sleep, don't even think about shaving off a few dollars (or minutes) here: It's your tip for good service!

This book will change not just the way you sleep but also the way you *think* about sleep. Part of that is accomplished through the two dozen case studies I share in the chapters to follow—success stories from my actual patients (names have been changed) with sleep challenges similar to those you might face now. You'll meet real people suffering from sleep disorders both rare and familiar—including snoring, insomnia, and sleep apnea—and learn how I came to help them when they had almost given up all hope.

Patients like Audrey, the concert violinist who taught at a prestigious university's school of music, who had suffered from insomnia for years and taken increasing amounts of prescription medications with no consistent success. Or Sam, the otherwise healthy general surgeon working long hours who came to see me because his snoring was so.thunderous, his wife had relegated him to the couch. Or Vivienne, whose strange behavior of unknowingly shopping in her sleep— for $7,000 pairs of designer shoes that were not even in her size (!)—was brought on by the high doses of sedatives she took to correct her insomnia. The expensive problem was depleting both her sleep bank *and* her bank account!

And I'll never forget Mark—an electrician who hadn't slept well for *15 years* after being diagnosed with severe obstructive sleep apnea and fitted with a CPAP (continuous positive airway pressure) device (which he hated, by the way). After seeing three sleep doctors, participating in three sleep studies, and even undergoing a few difficult surgeries to correct the problem, he was still struggling when he showed up in my office. Thankfully, I was finally able to help him (you will learn how in chapter 9)—and he now sleeps peacefully for the first time in over a decade. These are just a few of the many examples I share with you in this book.

Those of you with a history of difficult sleeping may have a hard time looking forward to bedtime. I get it, and I see that in my patients all the time. With that in mind, I also aim to transform the way you feel when those first rays of early morning sun stream in through your window. This book will help you embrace (and dare I say love?) sleep again and show you how to form positive associations with night settling in.

It will give you a new appreciation for sleep, which is available for free to all of us.

No matter your age, this book will help you revolutionize your patterns on a daily basis and support you on a renewed journey toward better sleep, better health, and ultimately a better life—not just for tonight but for a lifetime. This is especially relevant now that we've experienced the COVID-19 pandemic, when professional and personal stressors negatively impacted our sleep, thereby throwing off our sleep rhythms and weakening our immune systems, leaving us even more vulnerable to the virus. (Turn to chapter 8 for more on the pandemic's global impacts on sleep.)

And so here I find myself yet again "knocking" on doors (in a way) with this book, hoping to bring preventive health awareness to my readers, educate the masses, push the field to more prominence, and inspire the next generation of bright minds. Except this time, instead of evangelizing the benefits of polio eradication, it's sleep. For me, it always comes back to sleep.

You have 13.5 million shots at an amazing transformation. Are you ready to *really* sleep . . . and wake up to your dream life?

Dr. Abhinav Singh
Sleep Vigilante

PART I:

Unlocking the Secrets of Sleep

Chapter 1

Sleep: An Enduring Mystery

Sleep Vigilanteism: Show me something with better terms and conditions for the consumer than sleep.

Transforming Night into Day

No one realized it at the time, but at precisely 3 o'clock on September 4, 1882, one of sleep's greatest enemies bolted into the world.[1]

That enemy, we now know, is artificial light. When Thomas Edison hit the switch for his Pearl Street power plant that late summer day, lighting up a single square mile in Manhattan for the very first time, he forever altered the way we live, work, travel, dine, entertain . . . and sleep.

Electric lighting now powers economies, illuminates cities, and lets us shoot hoops late into the night if we want to. But this dazzling invention also has a dark side (as enemies do): It suppresses melatonin, upends the circadian rhythm, and robs the body of sleep, one of the most precious life-giving biological processes we have. Except we didn't really know that until recently. We spent generations discounting sleep until around 2000 or so, when scientists finally clued into how essential sleep is to our brain health, to our hearts, to our overall health and well-being. We are still learning more every day.

In the past, people usually slept a predictable set of hours, unencumbered by glowing screens and bulbs. Before the dawn of billboards and blinking TVs, most of humanity lived and slept by the natural rhythm of a rising and setting sun. People woke and stretched at dawn and turned in after dark. President Abraham Lincoln (who reportedly had trouble sleeping, especially during the Civil War)[2] probably suffered from insomnia and worked late into the night by dim candlelight. The universal lack of light placed limitations on what we could accomplish in a day. And so our modern ancestors—post–Industrial Revolution and pre the discovery and mass commercialization of artificial light—generally luxuriated in an hour or more of sleep per night than we get now. (That's 365 more hours of sleep *per year*.)

Every single day, I witness the detrimental effects of artificial light on my patients. We work so hard every day to raise our families and find success in our work that before we know it, we have exchanged sleep for productivity and entertainment—but at a terrible cost.

Meet James,* one of my patients, a talented jeweler and watchmaker. People don't usually seek out help from a sleep doctor like me until they've tried everything, they're desperate, and nothing seems to work. And so often it's because

---

* Names have been changed.

somebody complains that they snore—as was the case with James.

Every night, James would go to bed at 10 p.m., but he'd toss and turn, miserably awake, staring at the clock until 2 or 3 a.m., only for the alarm to jolt him up at 6. He logged just three hours of sleep a night, and the severe lack had started to take its toll. When he came to me, he felt crummy all the time. He was constantly tired, but not sleepy. (There's an important distinction to be made here between tired and sleepy, which I will discuss more in this book.) James was anxious, depressed, and diagnosed with attention deficit disorder. He had chest pains and popped a cocktail of meds prescribed by his doctor to try to alleviate the whole host of health issues invading his body.

I soon learned why sleep evaded him night after night. You see, James worked with a high-end clientele, and the labor to produce and repair fine jewelry requires meticulous manual work that must be done by hand. Although his store closed at 7 p.m., in order to have the pieces ready the next day, he spent the last hours of his workday toiling under bright lights and peering through magnifying glasses. Instead of winding down when the sun set, he beautified sparkling rings and necklaces—and put immense strain on his eyes and brain. You simply cannot prepare your body for sleep when you spend your evening hours soaking up artificial light and straining your eyes.

After breaking it down together and rethinking his nightly pattern, we were able to reset his sleep routine once and for all, much like the plan you will learn about in chapter 10. He followed my advice and is doing so much better now. Once he rediscovered his body's natural ability to sleep, his health improved—and he got off a majority of his meds. The moral of the story is we all need sleep to heal, and your body will let you know if that daily essential healing is not taking place.

If you are holding this book in your hands, you know that high-quality, healthy sleep is in short supply. You also probably neglect it more than you should; we all do. For most of our lives, working instead of sleeping has been glorified. Resting instead of living is deemed lazy. Every single day we make culturally accepted choices that negatively impact our sleep. And those choices then cement into habits. Read emails until midnight? Of course. Watch movies till 2? Sure. Pull an all-nighter in the City That Never Sleeps? Can't wait!

Setting aside 8 to 10 hours every night for sleep feels old-fashioned, doesn't it? How will we get anything done if we sleep all the time? Even Edison, who was awarded more than 1,000 patents in his lifetime, reportedly referred to sleep as "a heritage from our cave days," according to bestselling author James Maas in his book *Power Sleep*.[3] Edison kind of had a point: On its surface, anyway, sleep doesn't really make sense. Until you look deeper.

Nature's Mistake ... or Nature's Brilliance?

Dr. Allan Rechtschaffen, one of the world's foremost sleep researchers (who passed away in 2021 at age 93), said in 1978, "If sleep does not serve an absolutely vital function, it is the biggest mistake the evolutionary process ever made."[4] Inside his sleep lab at the University of Chicago, he began to make some interesting observations. For one thing, he found that rats deprived of sleep died in about two to four weeks.[5]

Does evolution make mistakes? Let's think about babies for a moment. In the beginning, when you were born, you came preprogrammed, by nature, with two voluntary skills that were essential. One is the ability to eat—nobody taught you that—and the second is the ability to sleep. We've all seen babies sleep in the brightest and loudest of environments. Why did nature not take a chance on your mother or your family teaching you these two essential actions? They must have been so incredibly important to our existence.

Except...sleep does seem almost antievolutionary. Evolution says preserve and procreate. In other words, make more of your own, gather food, and don't get killed. Keep your species alive. When you sleep, none of this is taking place. For 8 to 10 hours a day, you're in a vulnerable position, unable to defend yourself or your immediate family from attack. And you're not eating when you're sleeping (except for those sleepwalkers among us known to raid the fridge in the wee hours of the night).

And yet all of us sleep. And we spend one-third—13.5 million minutes, hopefully—of our lives sleeping.

This isn't some special insanity reserved only for humans (like overthinking or dancing the Macarena). Most animals sleep in one way or another—or at least get by with a power nap. From aardvarks to zebrafish, clear across the animal kingdom, they sleep too (even insects!). Some animals sleep standing up; others snooze beneath ocean waves; some find their favorite burrow or roosting spot; others grab some shut-eye midair while flying. We all somehow take part in this universal restorative experience called sleep. And just like us, most animals and birds that live on land also experience REM sleep, the sleep phase where dreams take flight. (You'll learn more about REM in chapter 4 of this book.)

> Humans are the only animals who willingly delay sleep—even when we know doing so is not in our best interest.

Scientists have gained fascinating insights about sleep by studying manatees, seals, and cetaceans like dolphins, whales, and porpoises. Have you ever wondered how dolphins sleep? Like us, dolphins are mammals that breathe air—and they would drown if they stayed underwater for hours at a time to sleep. Dr. Jerome M. Siegel of the UCLA Brain Research Institute found that when dolphins sleep, only half of their brain sleeps at a time. The unusual adaptation, called unihemispheric sleep, means that if they are underwater at night, the left half of their brain sleeps while the right half stays awake to do breathing runs. Then halfway through the night, it switches.

Thanks to unihemispheric slow-wave sleep, these particular ocean-loving mammals—who, like us, also sleep about eight hours a day—stay awake just enough to get their breath and remain vigilant with one eye open. It's the same idea with migratory birds, which fly for thousands of miles and are still able to navigate while sleeping. In contrast, it is believed that we humans experience bihemispheric sleep.

Melatonin, perhaps the most well-known sleep hormone, assists both animals and humans with their sleep cycles. As humans, we are designed to sleep at night. As evening settles in, the darkness jumpstarts our body's natural production of melatonin, signaling our biological night and preparing us for sleep. But what about mice, bats, and other nocturnal creatures, which are more active at night? It's the opposite! Nocturnal animals are activated (instead of relaxed) by melatonin. And so they—like my beautiful cats, Millie and Leo—wake up, run around, hunt, and play as night falls. All this sleep also means that animals preserve energy because they spend the daytime hours resting instead of hunting.

The paradox of sleep is that in nature's mysterious way, it aids in our survival while simultaneously rendering us helpless because of it. And we're only just beginning to wake up to its importance.

> To avoid becoming a feast for predators, it is believed that wild giraffes only need about 2 to 3 hours of sleep per day split into several parts. Meanwhile, a 1996 landmark study of giraffes in a zoo setting—where they do not need to hide from predators—found that these gentle giants sleep in fragments adding up to 4.6 hours per day.[6]

Who Cares about Sleep, Anyway?

Part of why scientists and clinicians like myself know so little about sleep is that even as modern medicine matured, sleep was a neglected field of study. Consider, for example, the groundbreaking discovery of insulin in 1921, which dramatically improved the life-span of a person with diabetes. Then in 1928, penicillin, the first antibiotic, was discovered, revolutionizing modern medicine globally following its development and distribution in the 1940s. These discoveries were made about 100 years ago (as of the printing of this book)—whereas "dream sleep" was only just discovered in 1953![7] But how could we have missed something so important to our health for so long? We've still just barely cracked the chapter on sleep. Why? As it turns out, multiple factors were at play.

The prevalence of sleep biases. In the 1980s, former UK prime minister Margaret Thatcher supposedly said, "Sleep is for wimps," an attitude perhaps shared by former Yahoo! CEO Marissa Mayer (a.k.a. Google's 20th employee), known for working 130-hour weeks.[8] According to the International Churchill Society, former UK prime minister Winston Churchill led Britain to victory in World War II by working feverishly through the night but prioritized afternoon catnaps to catch up on lost sleep. Edison reportedly said in 1914, "There is really no reason why men should go to bed at all";[9] meanwhile, rival inventor Nikola Tesla was known to only sleep two hours each day.[10] Narendra Modi, prime minister of India, is said to work 20 hours a day[11]—which leaves little time for sleep. Even as recently as 2019, the comedian Steve Harvey said, "Rich people don't sleep eight hours a day"—and you can probably still find this motivational video of his online.

In our society, so many of us look up to wealthy, successful, and powerful leaders, CEOs, and other influencers. So if they largely dismiss sleep as ineptitude or weakness, that ultimately impacts our attitudes and beliefs too.

Idolizing "the perfect soldier." Since the dawn of time, sleep has been a great weakness for being attacked. Throughout history's wars, enemies have been known to be killed while they slept, such as in the Paoli Massacre during the Revolutionary War, when sleepy, disoriented Patriot troops came under surprise attack by British soldiers. But during the 20th century especially, as technology evolved and allowed us to become more nimble in darkness, there emerged this idea of "the perfect soldier" who never fatigued, who could fight all hours of the day and night with minimal sleep. During the wars fought between 1900 and 2000, whoever conquered the night—and whoever developed the best weapons to aid the perfect soldier at night by land, sea, or air—claimed wartime superiority.

A lot of my patients have fought in combat, and I've seen firsthand what happens when we sell off sleep to gain this wartime advantage. War vets suffer mentally and physically upon return—and their sleep takes a real hit. My patients, some of whom fought in Desert Storm and in Afghanistan, tell me stories of extreme sleep deprivation. Days are spent awake and fighting, but then at night, they're still almost half awake, frequently startled by nighttime bombings and shellings. As a result, their sleep suffers for months and even years after, even if they're not on active duty. Back home, they face the same distractions as us—social obligations, TV, social media, children interrupting sleep, and so on—with the added strain of their wartime experience. It's a tall order to be "the perfect soldier."

Technological limitations. Another roadblock to the advancement of sleep research was a basic lack of technology. It wasn't until the 1920s that German psychiatrist Hans Berger had the idea to attach electrodes to a person's head to measure brain waves. For the first time, we witnessed electrical activity. He didn't know what it meant—and it remains a mystery still, a century later. And then in the 1950s, in a similar fashion, researchers started discovering sleep waves.

But measuring these kinds of data in the predigital era was a burdensome exercise. Everything had to be recorded on paper—reams and reams of paper consumed night after night. Just imagine for a moment trying to conduct a brain wave study with hundreds of participants, for eight hours each per night, and the resulting mountains of paper scientists had to dive and sift through to identify similarities and analyze the results.

Back then, sleep research wasn't just time consuming—it was also unglamorous. And think about it: Why would anyone want to dedicate their life to studying sleep, a wasteful pastime of the lazy and unmotivated? Of course, some scientists felt that passion and followed their hearts, though they didn't have a lot of company. It's a small circle even today: According to the American Academy of Sleep Medicine, as of 2017, there were just 7,500 board-certified sleep specialists in the United States.[12] I'm fortunate that I'm a member of this group. And of that group, only about 2,000 are granted fellowship into the American Academy of Sleep Medicine for their distinguished contribution and service to the field. I'm honored to be a member of this club too.

Things are changing for the better: Now we can record that information digitally and access results more easily. We can gather, analyze, and transport data as needed. And so, since the 1990s, a real upswing in sleep research has taken place. (See "The Sleep Discovery Timeline" for a year-by-year view of advancements in the past century.)

THE SLEEP DISCOVERY TIMELINE:
LANDMARK DISCOVERIES IN SLEEP

YEAR	DISCOVERY
1924	German psychiatrist Hans Berger discovers brain waves
1953	REM sleep discovered at the University of Chicago
1965	Discovery of sleep apnea[*]
1970	William Dement, one of the founding fathers of sleep medicine, opens the world's first sleep-disorders lab at Stanford University in California
1972	The discovery that snoring disrupts oxygen levels and blood pressure
1993	National Center on Sleep Disorders Research established, elevating loss of sleep to national health concern
2005	Lack of sleep correlates with a reduced ability to regulate blood sugar[†]
2013	Discovery that toxins are flushed from our brain as we sleep[‡]
2017	Discovery of the genes that control our sleep-wake cycle (circadian rhythm) wins the Nobel Prize
2018	Sleep loss correlates with more beta-amyloid in the brain (linked to Alzheimer's)[§]
2019	Delta waves during sleep solidify our long-term memories[‖]

[*] Richard Jung and Wolfgang Kuhlo, "Neurophysiological Studies of Abnormal Night Sleep and the Pickwickian Syndrome," *Progress in Brain Research* 18 (1965): 140–59, https://doi.org/10.1016/S0079-6123(08)63590-6.

[†] K. Spiegel, K. Knutson, R. Leproult, E. Tasali, and E. Van Cauter, "Sleep Loss: A Novel Risk Factor for Insulin Resistance and Type 2 Diabetes," *Journal of Applied Physiology* 99, no. 5 (November 2005): 2008–19, https://doi.org/10.1152/japplphysiol.00660.2005.

[‡] L. Xie et al., "Sleep Drives Metabolite Clearance from the Adult Brain," *Science* 342, no. 6156 (October 18, 2013): 373–77.

[§] E. Shokri-Kojori et al., "β-Amyloid Accumulation in the Human Brain after One Night of Sleep Deprivation," *Proceedings of the National Academy of Sciences* 115, no. 17 (April 24, 2018): 4483–88, https://www.pnas.org/doi/full/10.1073/pnas.1721694115.

[‖] CNRS, "A New Discovery: How Our Memories Stabilize While We Sleep," ScienceDaily, October 18, 2019, http://www.sciencedaily.com/releases/2019/10/191018125514.htm.

Misperceptions about snoring. Our lack of understanding about sleep also fed into false narratives that still prevail today. Look around at all the advertisements, cartoons, movies, and other imagery that has always surrounded sleep—think back from your childhood all the way up to now. In all of these images, snoring is universally depicted as a marker of deep, restful sleep when in fact the exact opposite is true. Can you believe we had it backward this whole time? And so now we have an entire society worldwide that accepts regular, chronic snoring as a common and normal (though slightly annoying) activity. The unfortunate reality is that snoring can indicate a whole array of serious health conditions and should be addressed.

All of this taken together over the past 150 years or so really was a perfect storm. From this idea of "the perfect soldier," to world leaders and celebrities commonly discounting or even bashing sleep, to technological obstacles and even cultural misperceptions about our basic understanding of snoring—we can finally try to understand why most of humanity lacked any desire to study or learn about what I believe may be *the* most important and underrated pillar of our health. Fifty years from now, we will look back and say, "Jeez, we slept on it for 200 years when we had the tools to get it right."

A Dream Come True

In this moment, we are finally on our way to getting it right. And that's partly why I felt so impassioned to write this book from the perspective of an MD who helps people like you every day. But even outside of my busy clinic in Indiana, sleep scientists are actually grabbing headlines now thanks to landmark discoveries happening at a fast pace. For example, the 2017 Nobel Prize in Physiology or Medicine went to three circadian rhythm biology researchers who discovered the molecular mechanisms controlling the sleep-wake circadian rhythm and how it helps us adapt to Earth's revolutions.

Plus, numerous celebrities and pop-culture icons—from Ariana Huffington and Gwyneth Paltrow to LeBron James and Tom Brady—are finally starting to speak out about the vital role sleep plays in their lives and share how it impacts their happiness, creativity, performance, and success. Sleep is starting to feel cool, especially in mainstream pop culture, for the first time in forever.

How did we get here? How did we jump from everyone universally discounting sleep to people excitedly talking about this life-giving biological function that we still don't fully understand?

One aspect we never lost sight of on this journey is our curiosity about dreams. It's the only aspect of sleep that never lost its glamour. We know that Aristotle philosophized about sleep and dreams in ancient Greece. More than 2,000 years later, Sigmund Freud published his theories in *The Interpretation of Dreams* (1899). Dreams captivate us. They always have, and they probably always will. Ever since ancient times, we have wanted to understand the inner workings behind them. (Stay tuned, because scientists are still trying to solve this mystery.)

Dreams are these bizarre, realistic-feeling visions where we see our dead relatives. We get chased by monsters or solve insurmountable problems. Sometimes we dream of the mundane, with no obvious meaning attached; other times, our dreams are grand in scale. My friend once experienced, in vivid detail, an entire pregnancy and raised a child for its first five years of life—in the span of a single night's dream. Yes, she was quite sad when she woke up.

We all experience dreams—about three to five a night, though many are quickly forgotten upon waking—and so the topic fascinates us endlessly. The pursuit for answers naturally led us here, to our modern discoveries of sleep. After World War II ended and we had more time on our hands, researchers finally began to devote more time to subjects like sleep, dreams, the effects of sleep deprivation, and so on. The discovery of REM sleep (where dreams materialize) in the 1950s was fun and weird at the same time. But all of these discoveries happened in a lab; nobody connected sleep to health.

Now we know better: Sleep is serious business. Since the 1990s, so many interesting discoveries have reshaped our views on sleep and turned everything we thought we knew on its head. So many unanswered questions continue to linger: What happens during sleep? What do these brain waves mean? Can you alter them? Can you enhance them? We do know that sleep (or the lack of it) impacts our health in so many surprising ways: our blood sugar levels, our risk of Alzheimer's, the health of our immune systems, unwanted weight gain, our heart health, our anxiety levels, and how prone we are to accidents. The list goes on and on—and scientists are just getting started.

CELEBRITY SLEEP TIMES: WHO GETS IT RIGHT?

4 hours

   Madonna

4–6 hours

   Bill Clinton

   Martha Stewart

5–6 hours

   Richard Branson

   Lucy Liu

6 hours

   Elon Musk

7 hours

   Bill Gates

Five 90-minute naps per day

   Cristiano Ronaldo

8 hours

   Deepak Chopra

   Ariana Huffington

   Lin-Manuel Miranda

   Venus Williams

8–9 hours

   Jane Fonda

10 hours

   Gwyneth Paltrow

11–12 hours

   Roger Federer

12 hours

   LeBron James

15 hours

   Mariah Carey

Sources: As reported in major media outlets. Approximate and subject to change.

The takeaway? Poor sleep equals poor health, which means a reduced life-span in terms of both quality and quantity here on beautiful Earth.

The next decade will yield an explosion in scientific discoveries because sleep touches everybody. From the cat, to the infant, to the finest soldier, everybody is at risk for sleep loss. Just as a pandemic spares no one, no one is immune from the effects of sleep deprivation: rich, poor, man, woman, healthy, sick, old, young.

This interconnectedness of sleep to whole-body health and wellness for all of humanity certainly woke me up—not just because I'm a sleep physician but also because of my background in internal medicine and deep interest in preventive medicine. Sleep is special because it's accessible to every single one of us. We should all be protecting our sleep. The good news is, transforming your sleep is achievable and something we can all do. I will show you exactly how to do it in this book.

Step inside Your Personal Sleep Elevator

Before you turn to chapter 2, which takes a closer look at the problems that arise within not just yourself but also our society at large when sleep deprivation sets in, I want to leave this idea with you.

Think of sleep as your personal sleep elevator. This elevator has eight floors, where each floor represents one hour of sleep. The last three floors (the last three hours of sleep) are the most essential—but the rule is, you must first pass through floors one to five to reach the top; you cannot skip.

Imagine that the first five floors represent essential functions: toxin removal, muscle and body repair, and other necessary maintenance and restoration chores. Floors six to eight are where emotions get managed, creativity blossoms, dreams unfold, memories get archived, neuroplasticity takes place. Believe me, you don't want to stop early and miss those floors!

But so many of us do. Some of us battle with insomnia or stressful jobs that steal our sleep. Creative people—like artists, musicians, and writers—are notorious for not getting enough sleep. Yet those final two to three hours are the most enriching. Those of us who only pass through the first five floors in the sleep elevator at night are missing out on all the important benefits of the last three. The goal of this book is to help you ride your sleep elevator to the top every single night. You will feel your best—and your health will thank you too.

Chapter 2

The Hidden Truths of Sleep Loss

*Sleep Vigilanteism: Sleep lost is sleep
lost. You cannot get it back.*

When I was just a child, long before I ever decided to embark on sleep science as my life's work, the devastating effects of sleep deprivation affected my life in a personal way. And it wasn't just my life—my family, and even much of my extended community at large in India at the time, also felt this impact.

That's the unfortunate truth about sleep loss: The consequences affect all of us, and no one is immune. And sometimes, when a chain of events goes terribly wrong, sleep deprivation can impact thousands of us in a single moment.

I can still recall the cold winter morning of December 3, 1984. I was just five at the time, a few days shy of my sixth birthday. I remember that an unusual phone call came in for my father, and I vividly recall him hastily packing a bag and rushing off to work. My stomach fluttered because I knew, even at such a young age, that something big must have gone wrong.

At the time, we lived in Itarsi, a key railway hub in the central Indian state of Madhya Pradesh. My father worked as a senior divisional mechanical engineer for Indian Railways, and he was a first responder of sorts. When my father jumped into a Jeep with some junior officers and took off for Bhopal, the state's capital about 100 kilometers north, they had no idea they were speeding straight into ground zero of one of the world's worst industrial disasters of all time.

My father had been told by headquarters in New Delhi that the trains weren't moving, that a special train of officials for Indian Railways was stuck, and to go "figure it out." This was way before cell phones, and no one yet knew the magnitude of what had happened.

He and his team drove straight to the Bhopal train station and realized something was very, very wrong. An eerie silence surrounded them. Dead cows with swollen stomachs lined the roads. He began coughing. His eyes burned. A horrible stench hung in the air. Someone finally informed them of a massive chemical leak, and he brought food to the stranded officials. Somehow they got the trains moving again, and he drove back home to us later that night once additional support arrived. He had quite the story to tell.

Soon we'd all come to learn that at around midnight on December 3, as most of the city slept, approximately 45 tons of highly toxic methyl isocyanate gas leaked out of the Union Carbide pesticide factory, blanketing 25 square miles. Though we don't know exact figures, more than 5,000 people likely perished in the immediate aftermath, and the staggering final death toll grew to at least 15,000.[1] More than 500,000 suffered debilitating injuries ranging from paralysis to chronic bronchitis.[2] Though the exact cause behind the Bhopal gas tragedy remains uncertain, it was later determined that mistakes by tired, overworked employees played a role. My father was one of the lucky ones: His cough went away after a short while.

Signs You Are Sleep Deprived

We all know that mistakes happen when we're sleep deprived. It could be as simple as clumsily dropping a coffee mug on the floor or as serious as crossing the median and inadvertently killing someone. So many accidents like these are preventable, but only if we, as a society and on a personal level, decide to take sleep more seriously—and sleep *loss* even more seriously.

So let's talk a little bit about the warning signs of sleep loss. There's more to this issue than you might think. So many of my patients who think they're getting plenty of sleep are surprised to learn that they actually aren't at all!

Consider my patient Will, a car mechanic who came to me miserably tired but initially told me he slept 7.5 hours a night: bed at 11 p.m., wake up at 6:30 a.m., then snooze till 7. Sounds good, right? Well, yes—except he was exhausted and foggy during the day. And once I started asking more questions and digging deeper, I realized why.

So many of us think we are getting the sleep we need. We're in bed for seven or eight hours; doesn't that count? Well, not necessarily. Will said he went to bed at 11. But it takes the average person at least 20 minutes to fall into the deep, restful state of sleep and 10 minutes to wake up. That's 30 minutes lost right there. Then when you snooze, you're not actually sleeping, and it's not helpful to your body: You're just hovering somewhere between wakefulness and sleep. So now Will's 7.5 hours actually log in at 6.5. Then Will shared with me that he wakes up twice a night to use the bathroom. So subtract another 20 minutes for each of those to get back into a restful state of sleep. Now he's down to about 5.5 hours, which is not enough rest and healing for mind-body wellness.

Will had been doing this night after night and then sleeping in on weekends. Except he just couldn't catch up. He felt so terrible, in fact, that his general doctor ended up checking his thyroid and poking and prodding for various other maladies and even prescribing pills when all he really needed to do was fix the "simple" problem of sleep deprivation. I gave him a plan and told him to try it for three weeks. Three weeks is all you need to get your sleep schedule back on track. Will followed my guidance and ultimately felt much better.

> Imagine driving on a bad road filled with potholes for five days and then on a good road for two days. Does the damage to your car get undone? It doesn't—and it's a similar scenario when you sleep poorly during the week and try to sleep in on weekends.

Why three weeks? It's not a random figure: Three weeks is the magic spot—the scientifically proven length of time it takes to rewire your brain and learn a new habit. And so if you experience the rewards of optimal sleep over three weeks, you are going to feel motivated to repeat that behavior. Try it for yourself and you'll see.

There are two kinds of sleep deprivation: acute and chronic. (Will suffered from chronic.) Acute sleep deprivation happens when you know you're supposed to go to bed, but you don't. Instead, you stay up late studying for a test, working the late shift, or staying out to celebrate with friends, for example. Acute sleep deprivation happens when you keep pushing through even though you know you really shouldn't. Your body reacts negatively in various ways, such as through duller reflexes, longer response times, higher blood sugar, increased heart rate, and impaired cognition and decision-making.

Your body tries to warn you too. Common signs you need more sleep include the following:

- head won't stop nodding
- bags under your eyes
- falling asleep the second your head hits the pillow
- lacking energy for normal daily tasks
- inability to keep your eyes open
- drifting into another lane while driving
- waking up tired
- excessive yawning
- falling asleep during meetings
- feeling overly irritated

What sets acute apart is that with this kind of sleep deprivation, you know you need sleep. And it happens after a week or less of sleep loss.

Don't Try This at Home

The longest documented time a human has tried to stay awake is 11 days and 25 minutes, when 17-year-old Randy Gardner broke the world record of going without sleep for a school science project in 1964. What happened? He slept for 14 hours afterward and then resumed his normal life with seemingly no ill effects. But he reportedly suffered from insomnia in later years.[3]

When an Acute Problem Becomes Not So Cute

The more dangerous type, I feel, is chronic sleep deprivation. Chronic sleep deprivation gets really ugly over time, and you don't actually know it's happening—until someone like me performs a clinical evaluation and figures it out. These are the people who regularly sleep between the hours of midnight to 6 a.m. They haven't reached the top floors of their sleep elevator in weeks, months, or even years. They think they've adapted to less sleep and that's all the sleep they need, but they haven't. And perhaps not surprisingly, the mind-body effects that set in with chronic sleep deprivation are much more severe.

You probably don't even know the following health issues could be sneaking up on you or someone that you love that is sleep deprived. But because I want you to understand the detrimental effects of chronic sleep loss, take a look at what sleep science has discovered.

Behavioral issues. We all know this from personal experience, don't we? From kids to adults, if you don't sleep well, you're signing up for being irritated, grumpy, hangry, and annoying. I could go on and on. You know immediately how you feel the next day when you've slept poorly, correct? And so many of us then take those feelings out on our spouse or kids or coworkers, which leads to relationship discord. Not good at all. It's also well established that chronic poor sleep leads to a whole host of mental health conditions, including anxiety, attention deficits, and depression.

Suboptimal performance. Depending on where you work, your company probably expects you to work really hard. They want to see you being productive, efficient, and creative 150 percent of the time. But as I discuss more in chapter 3, poor sleep takes away from that. You're drowsy at your desk and not able to focus well. You're forgetting important tasks. From the best athletes to the more common folk, everybody needs an adequate quantity and quality of sleep to perform at their best. Sleep is not a "can have." It is a nonnegotiable "must-have." For all of us.

Think of it this way: You know how you charge your phone at night so that the battery says 100 percent in the morning? Sleep works much the same way. Depriving yourself of sleep is like trying to work through 100 percent of a day with only 80 percent (or less) of a battery.

Cognitive deficits. This is one of my favorites because of the exciting research behind it. One landmark paper that came out in recent years tells us that poor sleep equals poor cognition. You know, you forget stuff—important things, like your anniversary or a doctor's appointment or even your dog's name. And we are beginning to understand why. What happens to your brain when you get optimal sleep? It gets a "pressure wash" of sorts that removes all the built-up toxins from a hard day's work. We take a closer look at this in chapter 4, where I explain what's happening and why and how dementia and Alzheimer's may fit into the equation.

More accidents. As the Bhopal gas tragedy shows, fatal accidents are yet another dangerous consequence of sleep deprivation. It's more common than you think: Turn to the chart at the end of this chapter, "Major Disasters Linked to Sleep Loss," and prepare to have your mind blown. Not all accidents are fatal, but we know this happens, and people can get hurt or die. People running low on sleep are responsible for more mistakes and accidents in the workplace (about 274,000 per year according to research published in the *Archives of General Psychiatry*[4]): Tired and sleep-deprived surgeons amputate the wrong leg in a surgery, and sleepy drivers are more likely to crash a car.

Yes, car accidents are a big one: None of us want a drowsy driver in the next lane on our way to work. And yet according to the National Highway Traffic Safety Administration, an estimated 91,000 car accidents in 2017 involved drowsy driving, resulting in an estimated 50,000 people injured and around 800 deaths. When you miss out on too much sleep, your reaction times are delayed, and it's hard to keep your eyes open. You just can't respond to emergency situations fast enough because your reflexes are blunted and your reaction times are increased.

Same thing with train accidents: Every year, it seems a train derailment on the East or West Coast can be traced back to sleep loss or an undiagnosed sleep disorder like sleep apnea, leading to unnecessary deaths. Although the National Transportation Safety Board has called for mandatory sleep apnea screening of train operators for years, in 2017, the federal government decided to abandon a proposed plan to require such regulation.[5] The move also included bus and truck drivers.

Unfortunately, sleep apnea can be deadly if not diagnosed and treated, especially if the sufferer is operating any kind of moving vehicle. I remember a married couple coming in to see me recently. The wife told me how he would nod off while she was in the passenger seat, and she had to whack him with her purse every time he veered off into the rumble strip. She was convinced he was trying to kill her to cash out her life insurance! Luckily, I was (hopefully) able to reassure her: No, he isn't trying to kill you. He has sleep apnea.

Weaker immunity. Sleep loss also affects your immune system. You may have heard experts talking about this during the COVID-19 pandemic. Your immune system functions less optimally when you sleep poorly, and you have a four times higher risk of catching a viral infection like the common cold. Another recent paper found evidence of the damage sleep deprivation causes on a cellular level.[6] Mitochondria, for instance, are your battery packs in every single cell you have. White blood cells are your soldiers, the frontline defense in your blood. Your white blood cells have less mitochondrial DNA if you are chronically sleep deprived. Which means your soldiers don't have enough energy to fight. Guess what that means? You're going to get sicker, you're going to stay sicker longer, and your recovery is going to take longer.

The Four Ds of Dangerous Driving

Most people are educated about the dangers of drinking and driving, as well as driving while under the influence of drugs, but what about the other two deadly Ds? One is distracted driving, which only recently gained widespread awareness after several states enacted laws banning the use of cell phones while driving.

The very last D refers to drowsy driving. Did you know that sleep deprivation actually leaves you *more* impaired than if you had consumed a few glasses of wine? This pivotal research was done by Dr. Drew Dawson and Dr. Kathryn Reid. (Dr. Reid was part of the faculty in the sleep lab at Northwestern when I trained with Dr. Zee.) Their drowsy driving studies show that participants awake for 17 hours exhibit even worse performance impairments compared to someone with a blood alcohol level of 0.05 percent.[7] After 24 hours, the awareness and response times of a sleep-deprived person match someone with a blood alcohol content of 0.10 percent. This is pretty scary when you realize that 1 in 25 adult drivers report having fallen asleep at the wheel sometime in the past month.

Although we have laws against drunk driving, we didn't have any against drowsy driving until New Jersey's Maggie's Law, named for a college student killed in a head-on collision in 1997 after a driver who hadn't slept for 30 hours veered across three lanes of traffic. Because there was no law on the books at the time of the accident, the driver got off with just a small fine.

Championed by her mother, Maggie's Law now makes driving a car after being awake for 24 hours a criminal offense. Arkansas enacted similar legislation in 2013.

With very few laws related to drowsy driving—and no laws addressing the serious problem of chronically sleep-deprived drivers (even years after Dr. Dawson and Dr. Reid's research)—society unfortunately remains behind the times when it comes to drowsy driving. I hope someday we decide to address this issue. The safety of your morning commute (and that of those you love) relies on the quality of sleep the previous night of all the drivers on the road rushing around you.

Weight gain. Weight gain is hugely tied to sleep. Why? When you sleep less, your stomach releases more of a hormone called ghrelin. That word sounds like "growling," doesn't it? Well, it does growl. This hormone sends a message to your brain, which screams, "E-A-T. Eat! Eat more! I'm not done!" And the hormone leptin, which says, "Stop eating, I'm feeling lean, I'm satisfied," is suppressed. So when you sleep less, you're signing up for more weight gain. Second, studies have shown that healthy adults, when they were made to sleep five or fewer hours a night, in just four weeks developed the patterns of prediabetes and insulin resistance. Think about that: This happened in four weeks to healthy adults with no other issues!

Cardiac problems and heart attacks. People started listening a little bit more when the connection between sleep loss and heart conditions was discovered. In the '90s, we learned that chronic poor sleep leads to hypertension. And so much more has been discovered in the last 20 years. For instance, there is a 300 percent higher calcification in the coronary arteries of healthy adults who sleep less. You read that right: 300 percent. Imagine that! You can think of sleep as your water softener, which may prevent this buildup. So when you sleep poorly, you're throwing your water softener right out the window. This allows calcium to build up in your vital cardiac plumbing, causing blockages and the potential for heart attacks.

Mortality. That's the cold, hard truth. The only truth in life is death. And sleeping less—five hours or less per night—equals a faster death. Otherwise healthy adults have a threefold higher chance of dying within six years of chronic poor sleeping of fewer than five hours a night.[8] And when you look at all the common sleep disorders—including sleep apnea, which involves snoring and breathing pauses at night—they're all linked to increased mortality. People who continue to ignore these problems can unknowingly shave off about 10 years of their life. *An entire decade.*

This isn't all just bad news. The good news is—and I hope you take this to heart—that fixing your sleep can likely fix a lot of this damage. It's not too late to try. I have even seen cardiac damage in patients get reversed, and once we improved their sleep, their hearts actually strengthened. It's so reward-ing to witness the transformation and watch them succeed with sleep therapy. For example, one patient of mine had a pacemaker, and he struggled with a failing heart working at only 25 percent capacity. Once we were able to get around his sleep problem and fix his issues like sleep apnea, his pump went up to almost 50 percent (55–60 percent at rest is con-sidered normal). That's significant because at 50 percent, you can ride a bike, play golf, and maybe get through a honey-do list. Just by attending to his sleep, he experienced such a qual-ity upgrade to his life. And you can too.

Think of it like this: You're not just saying, "Hey, I need to sleep a little better; I don't feel as good." You're saying, "I want to invest in my present and future health." Because the hidden health effects of sleep loss are expensive and detri-mental to your quality of life. Remember that mutual fund of 13.5 million I talked about in the introduction? Do you see the numbers adding up a little bit quicker now?

A "Public Health Problem"

The U.S. Centers for Disease Control and Prevention says that one-third of us don't get enough sleep. The organization also underscores sleep health's importance "for the public health of the nation." Clearly, they're right on point. If only we would listen!

You can imagine how this hurts our society at large when frontline workers, bus drivers, train engineers, pilots, air traf-fic controllers, or any other people in positions where they are responsible for another's well-being are sleep deprived. Even new parents, whose newborn keeps them up all night screaming, are at risk. And so when large numbers of us are collectively sleep deprived and not functioning at our peak at the same time, you can see how this ripples across society. You have impaired decision-making, more mistakes, less awareness, road rage, and even unhealthy people pushing past their limits on a larger scale—until eventually, their luck runs out. Just like what happened in 2015, when the nuclear submarine USS *Georgia* ran aground while pulling into port, causing $1 million in damages. It was later determined that a fatigued and sleep-deprived crew compromised safety and played a role in the accident.[9]

Everyone is at risk, whether you're in the military or a private citizen driving down the road. Overworked car-for-hire drivers are especially at risk for fatigue. They earn better rates at 4 a.m., so they're driving around all day and all night, and who knows when they slept last? These companies often require their drivers to take breaks after working for 12 hours, but that doesn't stop the driver from working for another rideshare company during that downtime.

I see a lot of commercial truck drivers who come in to get screened for disorders like sleep apnea, a typical requirement to renew their license. They walk into my office disgruntled and screaming and frustrated, fearful of losing their livelihood because of a potential diagnosis, but they usually come to understand that it's for their own health and safety—and ours. Those with sleep apnea that I've discovered and treated finally realize how much better they feel after we fix their sleep. The trucking company is happy too, because a single 18-wheeler accident involving a fatality can cost them an average of $1.5 million.

The thing most people don't realize is that whenever I look at sleep disorders, the entire family is affected. And then that damage spills so quickly into everything else—just like it did back in 1984, into the busy kitchen of my own home, when I was just a boy and the phone rang and I had to watch my dad rush off to handle a scary situation. Sleep disorders are underrecognized, underappreciated, and undervalued—and my life's passion will always be to change that line of thinking. I would love to create a domino effect where each of us asks one other person, "How did you sleep?" Valuing sleep and starting this conversation chain are so important. We need to talk about it more and help encourage one another. I expand on this idea a little more throughout this book.

Despite all the scientific findings out there, and even all the celebrities beginning to speak up about how precious sleep is, for the most part, our society still sees staying awake as some kind of trophy to win. I continue to see this misguided belief in many new patients too. People think, *If I work hard and sleep less, I can earn money, a higher position, accolades, and even boost my career.* But a lot of people don't see that all these health problems they're suffering from can actually be connected back to sleep. Hidden dangers connected to sleep loss do exist, and unfortunately, when you fail to protect against them, you're hurting yourself first—and then taking everyone else down with you.

There is no good barter with sleep loss. Eventually, you will pay it back—and with interest. The trade-in for sleep is very poor, and interest is very high on this loan. Sleep loss is like that rude collection agency that will come around and bang on your front door to collect. Nobody wants that.

MAJOR DISASTERS LINKED TO SLEEP LOSS

YEAR	DISASTER	ROLE OF SLEEP LOSS
1979	Three Mile Island[*]	Tired shift workers failed to notice a malfunction
1984	Bhopal gas disaster in India[†]	Night-shift performance failures
1986	*Challenger* explosion[*]	Sleep-deprived NASA managers
1986	Chernobyl[*]	Sleepy shift workers reacted too slowly
1989	Exxon *Valdez* spill[‡]	Ship's captain was asleep after a night of drinking
1999	American Airlines flight 1420 crash[§]	Captain had been awake for 16 hours
2010	Air India Express flight 812 crash[‖]	Captain snoring on the voice recorder

[*] M. M. Mitler et al., "Catastrophes, Sleep, and Public Policy: Consensus Report," *Sleep* 11, no. 1 (1988): 100–109, https://doi.org/10.1093/sleep/11.1.100.

[†] Institute of Medicine (US) Committee on Sleep Medicine and Research, H. R. Colten, and B. M. Altevogt, eds., *Sleep Disorders and Sleep Deprivation: An Unmet Public Health Problem* (Washington, DC: National Academies Press, 2006), 4, https://doi.org/10.17226/11617.

[‡] Final Report from the Alaska Oil Spill Commission, February 1990, State of Alaska, pp. 5–14.

[§] Beth Lewandowski, "Pilot Fatigue, Error Probable Causes of '99 Little Rock Crash," CNN, October 23, 2001, http://edition.cnn.com/2001/US/10/23/little.rock.crash/index.html.

[‖] Yara Q. Wingelaar-Jagt et al., "Fatigue in Aviation: Safety Risks, Preventive Strategies and Pharmacological Interventions," *Frontiers in Physiology* 12 (September 6, 2021): 712628, https://doi.org/10.3389/fphys.2021.712628.

Here's a crazy idea that you may not have thought about before: *Humanity as a whole will benefit from everyone sleeping better.*

We need to rethink sleep and make sleep sacred again. The entire world would be so much better if everyone slept eight hours a night. It would be like a utopia! People would be happier, healthier, more productive. That positivity, in turn, would flow into our society and make the world a better place. Optimistic? Perhaps. But I believe this to be true.

The best place to start is with yourself. I encourage you to keep an open mind when it comes to reframing sleep's importance in your life. My hope is that the next chapter, which spotlights sleep's integral connection to performance, success, and future possibility, will help you find and hold onto your inner motivation to sleep longer and better for a lifetime.

Chapter 3

The Sleep-Success Connection

Sleep Vigilanteism: Sleep is your health's shiniest vulnerability—and it's easier to tarnish than you think.

B ack when I first came to America to pursue my dream of studying medicine in the United States, I boarded my plane in India with three treasured possessions: a heart full of optimism, my acoustic guitar (a gift from my father), and my black embroidered Chicago Bulls hat. Little did I know (nor could I have ever imagined) that in about 20 years' time, I would become an official sleep doctor for an NBA team: the Indiana Pacers.

This exciting development transpired for me in the fall of 2021 while immersed in writing this book. And I am finding that people are still sometimes surprised when they hear that an NBA sports team has a sleep physician on staff. An orthopedic surgeon, sure, but a sleep doc? What?

It makes sense when you consider how our knowledge of sleep science has accelerated in recent years, even though I still consider this a newer field of study. Think about it: A pro athlete's exercise is taken care of. So is their nutrition—a nutritionist travels with the team, measuring meals and ensuring proper hydration and nutrition. Those two pillars of health are covered. But outside the court or training facility, things can get a little tricky—yet that third pillar, sleep, is just as important as the other two when it comes to performance. When the players finally pull into their driveways at the end of a long day and close the doors behind them, sleep becomes this unsupervised action left to the individual player's discretion. Some players do well in protecting their sleep; others not so much. Problems creep in when sleep is not properly managed.

My work with the players focuses on helping them embrace this idea that sleep and success are interlinked. Exceptional sleep makes your whole body stronger: It helps your body repair muscles; it gives your immune system a boost; and it makes you a faster and, I believe, better player on the court. Every major sports team hopes their elite athletes can find that special edge—the one that means the difference between winning a two-foot-tall, 15.5-pound golden trophy and *almost* winning it (but not quite). Sleep can give you that edge.

At the same time, all of us team doctors aim to protect the physical and emotional health of our players and staff to ensure everyone's in top-notch condition. Sleep optimization helps with that too.

And so now I find myself courtside during games and practices or back in the weight room, dressed in my official Pacers gear, fully badged, and on a mission: I want to get to know the players better, yes, but I also need to find ways to sell them on this idea that sleep must be an essential component of their daily training regimens. Multiple studies show[1] that athletes who sleep more than eight hours per night

- have more stamina for training;
- are less prone to injury;
- can power through longer before feeling fatigued;
- are more emotionally grounded and cognitively stable, so they can make strategic game-winning decisions (Should they take a three-point shot before the buzzer or not?);
- have improved accuracy (A 2011 Stanford study found that basketball players who slept 10 hours per night increased their accuracy in free throws by 9 percent.[2]);
- can move faster;
- have quicker reaction times; and
- have stronger immune systems and a lower risk for respiratory diseases and illnesses in general.

That all sounds great! Except here's the problem: How are professional athletes supposed to get eight hours of sleep every night? They endure sleep disruptions on an almost daily basis but are still expected to perform at peak ability. They train all day and then have to rush to another city for a game. They're these tall, muscular players stuck in an airplane at midnight, crossing time zones, and checking in and out of hotel after hotel.

Sleep is a habit situation, a rhythm. No human is at their most comfortable sleeping in an unfamiliar environment. You like the repeated environment of your own room, your own pillows. Maybe your child, pet, or partner has become part of your sleep environment and/or ritual, but everything keeps changing when you're on the road.

For pro athletes, healthy sleep of appropriate quality and quantity can elude them even if they're home. Maybe it's 11 p.m. and they're finally driving home, only to collapse on the couch before getting up early for a game, flight, media commitment, or practice session the next day.

Let's say they're home with their families, and maybe they unwind with their smartphone or TV or video games (like we all do, except screens—especially bright ones—are some of the worst sleep disruptors). They may nod off to sleep only to have their kids scream out, "Daddy! Daddy!" at 2 a.m. If they don't have kids, they may be up late partying with their friends.

Now add on top of this their emotional state: What if they didn't do well in that day's game? Here they are, charged with adrenaline, slammed with media interviews, stressed out, and feeling the weight of being scrutinized on social media, by coaches, by ESPN replays. They're exhausted, hungry, and maybe even injured; they've exerted themselves beyond human capacity. Now they really start to look superhuman, don't they? This is the life of an elite athlete, and the schedule simply does not allow a lot of room for regular, consistent sleep.

But it must. I'm still finding out if sleep health is a new concept for some of the players and if any of them take their sleep for granted. But even if they don't consciously neglect their sleep, the aforementioned stresses (and sometimes even a sleep disorder) take their toll. I see a fair amount of insomnia, circadian disruptions, excessive daytime sleepiness, and even snoring and sleep apnea in these pro athletes. Therefore, creating a plan, educating them, and above all, getting their buy-in are essential. It's all about being proactive with sleep interventions instead of reactive. I can already tell they want to learn: In my first two hours of meeting everyone on the team, several players and staff members came over and said, "Dr. Singh! I need to meet with you."

Even though all of us can benefit from better sleep—no exceptions—athletes must protect it even more because of everything that's at stake for them and their team, because they train and compete at such a high level, and because they push their bodies harder than most of us ever will. Imagine swimming for leisure versus swimming competitively. Competitive swimmers are going to need a longer rest period; their bodies ache for all the resources they can get to recover after that.

All pro athletes start out good, but few become great, and even fewer become legends. Tennis great Roger Federer reportedly sleeps around 12 hours a day; so does NBA champion LeBron James. The difference between a good athlete and a great one is how long their peak performance lasts. These guys still deliver the goods well beyond anyone else in their age group. They're doing something different than the others. Could winning at sleep be one of their secrets?

Here's a question for you. Have you ever wondered what would happen if you took your sleep as seriously as an NBA All-Star? How might your life transform?

Sleep Spotlight: Roy Hibbert, Two-Time NBA All-Star

I want to share with you an incredible story of sleep success from one of my patients, Roy Hibbert. (Roy has graciously allowed us to use his real name for this book.) You may already know him as a two-time NBA All-Star and a player for such teams as the Indiana Pacers, the Los Angeles Lakers, and the Charlotte Hornets. Most recently, he coached the Philadelphia 76ers—but he's decided to take a break now to become a stay-at-home dad and focus on his two young children. "To be honest, the coaches spend more time with the players and the staff than with their own family," he said when we interviewed him for this book.

I first met Roy back in 2013—before he made All-Star for the second time—after one of my partners at work got selected to be the official team internist for the Indiana Pacers. I was already educating all my partner physicians at work on my "360 degrees of sleep awareness" philosophy of sleeping better to live better, which I still share with anyone and everyone around me who will listen—patients, family, friends, neighbors, colleagues, my cats, my poor wife, even my plants sometimes, and even you now, as I share my life's passion in this book! And so before long, I noticed my partner adopting a lower threshold for sending NBA players and staff my way. He seemed more mindful that something as simple as sleep could be affecting their performance and general well-being.

One of those players was seven foot, two inch Roy, who, at the time, played the center position for the Pacers. "I always took my health very seriously," Roy said. "Eating right, lifting, working out. I was getting all that, but for some reason, I felt that I didn't have as many gains in the weight room as I should."

When he came to see me, he told me he was in bed at 10 p.m. and up at 8 a.m. That is an incredible 10 hours! But he still felt lethargic and like he was dragging through the day. Something was interfering with his sleep. The quantity seemed adequate, but could it be the quality?

"Some people told me in the past that I snored," said Roy. "My dad snored. I figured that's just what people do. I never knew it could be the result of something scientific. I thought it was my everyday normal. I thought it must have been food or being tired from working out so much."

I asked Roy to do an overnight sleep study in the sleep center, which isn't an easy request—especially when a person's schedule is as busy as his. "I had nodes put on me," Roy remembered. "I got there at 10 p.m. I had a hard time falling asleep but finally did. I slept, and they told me they got enough info."

Yes, we did: I discovered that Roy had sleep apnea. That explained his overwhelming fatigue during the day. I also learned that he could sleep better on the left side (but not the right). With the help of a sleep dentist, we ultimately fitted him with a mouth appliance (not to be confused with a bite guard) that moved his lower jaw forward because he wasn't ready to try CPAP therapy at that time. "Luckily, I talked to Dr. Singh," Roy said. "It's been a work in progress since then."

There are a few different approaches we take when treating sleep apnea, and it depends on the patient. Sometimes we try a mouthpiece. Other times we recommend a CPAP based on their severity, body type, and postural influence on sleep apnea. For some patients, if they are obese, they can try to lose weight and see if that helps. Roy wasn't overweight, and he wanted to try the mouth appliance first because it fit his comfort level at the time, especially considering his busy travel schedule.

I was so happy to hear that in just two days, he started to feel better. "I didn't feel like I needed that extra hour of sleep," said Roy. "I didn't have that anymore. I woke up and felt like I got enough sleep. I used to wake up groggy or wish I didn't have to get out of bed. Now I felt like: I'm ready to go!" Roy told me he felt more energized than he had in years, even though he was up early in the morning for practices, playing four games in five nights, and traveling city to city for games. He went on to have a very successful career after we treated him for his sleep disorder.

Fast-forward eight years, and Roy has since upgraded to a CPAP. You see, Roy was in his 20s when he first came to see me. He wasn't married, and he was a cool NBA player living the dream. He didn't even want to try CPAP therapy at that time. (I would like to note this is a common reluctance among my patients.) "I was 25 or 26 at the time," said Roy. "I didn't think wearing a CPAP was the coolest thing to do. I chose to go the other route with the mouthpiece. But as I got older and wiser, I decided to try the CPAP. I wish I had done that 10 years ago! Who cares what I look like as I'm sleeping?"

The problem with his mouthpiece was that he would grind his teeth at night and break it. Then he got clear aligners to straighten his teeth, and then the mouthpiece didn't fit at all, so he stopped using it for his sleep apnea. His sleep was starting to suffer, so he showed up in my office again. This time, Roy was in his 30s, settled, and much more open to trying something new. But adjusting to the CPAP wasn't exactly easy. I told him to keep trying it and assured him that it would get easier. "I had a tough time the first couple of nights," Roy said. I moved him to a bilevel PAP (positive airway pressure) device and taught him some breathing exercises, and he tells me "it's been smooth sailing" since then.

Roy was older now, and he was experiencing firsthand how he simply could not suffer through poor sleep anymore the way he did in his youth. We all realize this as we age. He just wishes the young up-and-coming NBA players could learn from his experience now because sleep optimization isn't always on their radar.

"As an older player, I used to see the young guys going out and enjoying life," Roy said. "I told them, make sure you get your rest—the other team is in bed getting their rest for the day. And when you're younger, you can get away with a lot more. As you get older, you can't skip sleep. You have to do it the right way."

Not to mention, "maybe there is a stigma about using CPAP," Roy said. "But if it can help you with games and be sharper on the court, it's worth it." Even Shaq has been diagnosed with sleep apnea and has done commercials to promote the CPAP apparatus that changed his life.

Now that he's a busy dad, Roy needs all the sleep he can get. "Consistency is key. When you have kids, they get up early. So I need to make sure I'm in bed so I have energy," Roy said, adding that when he doesn't get his sleep, he's grumpier and less patient. (Aren't we all?) He also knows that I want him to log a full 7 hours and 45 minutes every single night, no exceptions, and that I'm able to review his sleep data on my laptop. Roy has to think twice now before squeezing in that extra episode of the *Real Housewives of Orange County* on a Friday night with his wife. (I understand the temptation— I really do. But sleep should always come first!)

Successful People Need Sleep

NBA players aren't the only ones who need eight-plus hours a night. Everybody needs sleep, but I especially recommend it to the most successful among us, the people we might consider the rock stars in their field who are changing the world—the leaders and the creators, the luminaries and the visionaries, the disruptors and the game changers. Optimal sleep supports

- creativity,
- strategic decision-making,
- clarity,
- speed and efficiency of work,
- better judgment,
- improved focus,
- alertness,
- mood regulation, and
- even more.

Sleep is the secret weapon your competitors are probably not using (yet). Even better, the intellectual and emotional advantages that come from regular deep sleep will help you succeed in that make-or-break meeting with a client, or that upcoming pitch to an angel investor, or the big, sparkly idea you're hoping to bring into the world. Even billionaire entrepreneur Elon Musk, who didn't always make time for sleep in his past, told a podcast in 2021 that he needs to get around six hours a night at least or his productivity declines. (Don't miss chapter 5, where I've compiled all the beautiful benefits of sleep—50 of them—to help inspire you.)

I can tell you that I see high-profile patients with sleep problems all the time. They work at such an advanced level that when their sleep gets disrupted, they notice right away. Their normally stellar performance feels like it might falter, and that is a nightmare for them. High achievers simply cannot let that happen. In the medical field, I work with a lot of brilliant surgeons and other leading medical specialists who can't afford to feel less than perfect because patients' lives depend on their skill and attentiveness every single day.

Sam is one example. This otherwise healthy general surgeon / chief of staff came to see me because he felt he was so tired that he was slipping a notch. Sam was in his early 50s, successful, and in the prime of his career. After a diagnosis of sleep apnea, we fitted him with a custom mouthpiece (with the help of a sleep-specialized dentist), and he experienced the positive results right away.

I also worked with an exceptional gastroenterologist, a pioneer and leader in his field, who came to me because he was experiencing a severe case of OTC, or ouch to couch (coined by the Sleep Vigilante himself!). This unfortunate situation happens when the patient snores so loudly that their partner elbows them in bed at night, hoping that they roll over, reduce snoring, and stop disrupting their sleep.

Instead, they usually end up sleeping on the couch. Apparently, he was also kicking and twitching a lot at night, messing up the sheets and comforters and disrupting his wife. His OTC was bad, but even worse, he also experienced extreme daytime fatigue and sleepiness during the day (not a great feeling when you see a busy day ahead and a line of patients in your waiting room). Our sleep study showed prominent snoring but only mild sleep apnea, and his nighttime twitching events coincided with his bouts of snoring. I told him that once we treated him for his sleep apnea, it would all improve. He ended up choosing CPAP, and the right mask and pressure settings really worked for him.

Don't Become an Ouch Potato!

What is an "ouch potato," you ask? Well, you've become an ouch potato when your snoring is so bad you find yourself sleeping on the couch instead of in bed next to your partner.

Most snorers don't start out this way. There are three stages to becoming an ouch potato:

Stage 1: Ouch *or* Couch. In the beginning, your bed partner is more patient with you. They're not going to elbow you right away. But you know your snoring bothers them, so sometimes you go to the couch (before you get the elbow, ouch).

Stage 2: Ouch *to* Couch. Now the elbowing at night is becoming a repetitive thing while you're in bed with your partner, who simply can't take it anymore. And so you know every night, even if you start out in bed, it's three strikes (elbows) and then you're relegated to the couch.

Stage 3: Couch to Couch. You've neglected your snoring for a really long time once you reach this stage. You're not even in the bed anymore! Instead, you start out on one couch, then end up dragging your blankets to the other because this one's too lumpy. It's a bad situation all around: When you're sleeping this poorly, you've probably put on some extra pounds too. And you're missing out on snuggle time with your partner. Time to see your doc!

Outside the medical field, you have people like Frederik, the security detail chief for the CEO of a Fortune 200 global biomedical corporation. He had sleep apnea and already used a CPAP but came to me extremely fatigued and told me the machine wasn't working for him anymore. I soon learned he wasn't able to use it consistently because he traveled on planes all over the world, 15 days a month. The CPAP was too big to take with him, so half the time he just slept without it. (Not a good idea!) It was like taking one step forward and one back—with no progress being made. We found a smaller, portable travel CPAP with a battery pack that could be used on airplanes. It was a simple solution with life-changing results for this patient.

I encountered a similar situation with Dax, another patient of mine, who is the lead guitar tech for a world-famous, critically acclaimed, Grammy-winning musician. This guy was in his mid-40s and slogging through a grueling travel schedule that involved following the band as it zigzagged the globe. His work involved staying up late to "tear down" after a show and getting up early at the next venue for setup. He'd been extremely fatigued, was gaining weight, and had acid reflux—and then we discovered after a sleep study that his was also a hidden case of severe sleep apnea on top of chronic sleep deprivation. Just like Frederik, the security detail chief, Dax also had reservations and wondered how he was going to treat his sleep disorder when he was in and out of airplanes and hardly ever home. Again, we found a smaller device, got it on just the right setting for him, and off he went. He was sleeping great and better within weeks.

My high-profile patients often blame their careers for what they are feeling. The stress of their lifestyle is part of it, yes, but it often can be traced back to sleep deprivation, which could be in the form of quantity as well as quality deprivation. These individuals challenge themselves more than a lot of us do. They're highly competitive, comparing themselves to their peers. They come to me and say, "I have everything this guy has: the coaching, the motivation, the resources, the talent. Why am I not achieving the same?" It's true, they have it all: their IQ, their EQ (emotional quotient), and their $Q (dollar quotient)—but what they often overlook is their ZQ, or sleep quotient! And so I ask of them (as I ask of you right now too), "What's your ZQ?"

Quiz: What's Your ZQ?

Do you get amazing sleep, or could unknown sleep disruptions be hindering your sleep? Knowing your sleep quotient, or ZQ, is an important factor in determining the overall health and quality of your sleep. Take this quiz and find out if a visit with a sleep physician is in order.

Dr. Singh's DOZE Sleep Quotient Assessment

1. Do you frequently **desire** a nap in the day?
2. Do you wish you had more **oomph** during waking hours?
3. Do you feel you need to get more **Zzzs**?
4. Is your bed partner **exasperated** with your sleeping behaviors (snoring, restlessness, etc.)?

   Scoring: Any "yes" answer to the above questions warrants a chat with your health care provider or sleep physician. You may have a hidden sleep disorder and not even know it.

The Great Travel Unravel

These stories show a few things: First, a lot of people have sleep apnea and don't even know it until they come to see a specialist like me. Second, successful people work long hours in demanding jobs and sometimes even pull all-nighters—and if chronic sleep deprivation (quality and quantity) is present, it can interfere with their ability to perform at that high level long term.

Sleep Quality versus Quantity

Sleep quantity is what meets the eye: How many hours did you get last night? Sleep quality, by contrast, indicates how *well* you're sleeping. It doesn't meet the eye at all—it meets the ears of your bed partner, who's been listening to you snore for the past two hours. Or it meets your ribs when your partner elbows you to quiet down!

Often, sleep deprivation discussions stop at quantity, but they shouldn't. The number of hours you get each night matters, of course. But the *quality* of that sleep matters just as much.

Another common thread I see, especially among artists, musicians, pro athletes, and top-ranking executives, is this: Their jobs often demand that they live out of suitcases, rest on airplanes (good luck with that), and sleep in hotel rooms instead of their own beds. Frequent travel will unravel your sleep even if you usually sleep great, and the impacts on health, performance, and success cannot be overlooked. If this applies to you, just compare your sleep before and after March 2020. During the COVID pandemic lockdown, many of these kinds of jet-setters found themselves home for months on end and not using their passports for the first time in ages. As a result, many were able to rediscover their natural sleep rhythm and remember how good it feels. (See chapter 8, "While You Were Sleeping . . . during the Pandemic," for more on how COVID affected sleep worldwide—because although some improved their sleep during this time, for a lot of people, it just got worse.)

When your sleep rhythm gets upended, especially due to travel, you feel it. It's been documented that West Coast pro athletes perform better when traveling east compared to East Coast teams traveling west. If a game starts at 7 p.m. Eastern Time, the internal clock of a California athlete thinks it's just 4 p.m. They will play better and stronger even without home-court advantage thanks to their natural *circadian* advantage. Their body hasn't adjusted to the new time zone yet.

Now let's go the other way. When East Coast players fly west for a 7 p.m. game, their body acts like it's 10 p.m. Here they are on the court, and their melatonin is starting to release. Until they adjust to the new time zone, they are going to feel more tired than their competition, and studies do show that their performance suffers.[3] No sport is immune: The same goes for the NFL, the NHL, and so on. Kind of a bummer for East Coast athletes! (I'd like to point out that although the Pacers are based in the Midwest, here in Indianapolis, we're technically in an East Coast time zone. They do indeed face this challenge when they fly to the West Coast for games, and I will get to that soon.)

Crossing time zones messes up your circadian rhythm, your sleep, and your performance, no matter which direction you're headed, and it's worse the farther you go. You know this if you've ever experienced jet lag. (Travel two or more time zones, and you'll feel it.) The NBA knows it too, so they've enlisted people like me to help minimize the impacts on the players and support staff.

We know the players experience a circadian imbalance flying west, so what can we do? We can use tools and strategies tailored to each individual player to help them stay aware of and favorably align with their circadian rhythm and give them an all-important circadian edge.

Circadian edge: Achieving internal and external harmony and synchrony so that you can live strong, achieve your goals, and perform at peak level.

Pretty soon after I signed with the Pacers, they flew to Portland for a game. It was played at 7 p.m. local time, which was 10 p.m. Indianapolis time. Their melatonin was rising just as they were hitting the court. Do you think they were going to play their best? Nope. Despite leading by seven points in the fourth quarter, they still lost. Of course, every game played is layered and complex, but the impact of sleep loss is real. If we can move their body clocks closer to their peak *before* a game—which takes time—they can access that circadian edge and perform at a higher level.

Let's say the Pacers have a West Coast game on the calendar. I can work with each player individually ahead of time and tailor a specific plan for that athlete to help them maximize their circadian edge and, therefore, perform at their best no matter what city they're in. How is this done? It involves evaluating their current sleep pattern, making a plan, and implementing changes a few days in advance. It will require them to start taking melatonin prior to travel and gradually move their bedtimes and wake times by a few hours. When you get the formula just right, they'll adjust to the new time zone at a quicker pace, and the expected ill effects on their game will lessen.

Finding Your Own Circadian Edge

You may not be an NBA player with access to your own private sleep coach making sure your sleep is on point, but you can still learn how to use the circadian edge to your benefit.

First, you have to understand that sleep is a 24-hour deal. Sleep is not just snoozing under a fluffy duvet with an eye mask at night; it's also what you do during the day. When are your mealtimes? When are you exercising? When are your light exposures happening? What are you doing to train your body's circadian rhythm? The circadian system is a 24-hour clock that regulates our sleep-wake rhythms. Of the many circadian rhythms in the body, sleep-wake is a very important one. It is made up of an alerting signal during the day that works in tandem with a homeostatic drive to help promote sleep at night. It's while you are awake that you are actually building up your sleep drive. (More on this in the next chapter.)

In an ideal world, when you go to bed on time, sleep eight hours, and wake up feeling rested, everything works in harmony and synchrony, and you feel good. Optimizing your sleep on a daily, weekly, and monthly basis means you are keeping your circadian rhythm on key and in harmony. When it's working right, you're going to feel it with your mood, your patience levels, your concentration, your performance, your health, and so on.

The circadian edge can fit into your day-to-day life, or it can be tweaked for future travel. Your body performs differently at different times of day, and once you know that, you can try to schedule games or practices or meetings for specific times. How do you think teenage swimmers feel when their alarm clocks scream at them at 5 a.m. for swim practice? They feel horrible. But if you work *with* your internal body clock (instead of against it), you can plan practices at more harmonious times and adjust sleep times just so. Surprise: They perform better and achieve more when they do that.

Michael H. Smolensky, PhD, a pioneer in the field of clinical chronobiology, explained the 24-hour circadian clock in detail in his popular book *The Body Clock Guide to Better Health*, coauthored with Lynne Lamberg.[4] The book shows how different hours of the day correlate with your body's physiology and peak alertness, coordination, reaction times, muscle strength, and so on. If we were to adapt this concept researched by Smolensky and others to sports, business, or life (and keep in mind that some sports probably fall into more than one category), it might look something like the following Sample Schedule for Peak Performance.

Sample Schedule for Peak Performance

7 a.m.: Wake up

10 a.m.: Most alert—boxing, soccer, that important business meeting

2:30 p.m.: Best coordination of the day—basketball, hockey, volleyball, that important surgery

3:30 p.m.: Fastest reaction times—baseball, martial arts, racecar driving, tennis, flying an airplane

5 p.m.: Heart and muscles at peak strength—football, golfing, running, swimming

9 p.m.: Melatonin release begins

10 p.m.: Bedtime

2-4 a.m.: Window for deep sleep. I like to think of 4 a.m. as the temperature nadir and your Mariana Trench of sleep. (The Mariana Trench is the deepest point in the Pacific Ocean.)

4-6 a.m.: REM sleep in its most concentrated state happens here, which is especially important for creatives. So if you have a song you want to finish, you have a tricky problem you need to solve, or you're plotting the next bestseller, getting all your REM sleep will be crucial to you accomplishing your brightest ideas.

This is what your schedule might look like on a normal day. But remember, it can be pulled forward or back like I do with my traveling basketball players. Let's say you have to fly from New York to the UK next week for an important meeting. Just imagine for a second winging it and arriving in London for a 9 a.m. meeting, except you show up sleep deprived because your body thinks it's 4 a.m.—which is usually your time for deepest sleep. It's painful just thinking about it!

But if you take steps to minimize circadian asynchrony in advance, you can adjust faster and still bring your A game. Your jet lag will not be as severe, and you can get to enjoying your time in this new city faster.

Just like the pro athletes do, you can start a few days ahead of time by doing the following:

- Take ½ milligram of melatonin at specific times during the day (it depends on how many time zones you're crossing and which direction you're going).
- Soak up (or avoid) bright light exposure in the mornings and/or evenings.
- Gradually move your sleep and wake times to help you achieve alignment with the new time.
- For the custom specifics you'll need to make this work, talk to your doctor or a sleep physician once you know your travel details, or try a jet lag optimization calculator, which is easy to find online.

THE FOUR KINDS OF PREVENTION:
FROM GOOD TO BEST

1. **Primordial prevention:** This refers to having a plan *before* you have a health problem. In terms of sleep, it means following a plan and practicing better sleep habits now, even though there are no risk factors present or any signs of a disorder or health problem. Primordial prevention is the ideal scenario, and it's important to me because it fits into my "360 degrees of sleep awareness" philosophy. All people should invest in better sleep. Every single one of us, and everyone around us. Even if you think you sleep great now, you can always sleep better. The majority of this investment does not cost a thing; it just takes a little vitamin D—where D stands for discipline. With primordial prevention, you don't let your sleep drift—even for one night.

2. **Primary prevention:** This type of prevention occurs once a risk factor presents itself. Let's say you are diagnosed with high blood pressure. Primary prevention helps you get back on track so you can hopefully prevent a heart attack from occurring at all.

3. **Secondary prevention:** This is not my favorite kind, but we do implement it often. With secondary prevention, you are helping the person regain their health *after* the heart attack or regain their sleep after they've experienced chronic insomnia for five years.

4. **Tertiary prevention:** In this final stage, when interventions have not been as successful as hoped or when preventing the disease or condition is no longer an option, we aim to minimize complications and recurrences and improve the quality of life of the patient as much as possible.

Sleep Is a Sport

I encourage everyone (especially the Pacers!) to take their sleep seriously. Sleep can also be thought of as a sport, and the more you practice and invest time into it, the better you get at it. Just think, you could be a premier *slumber*jack of sleep!

When it comes to star basketball players, winning games is a great reason to care about a player's sleep schedule and circadian harmony, sure. But I also recognize the deeper implications: If athletes live, train, and play when chronically sleep deprived, their health suffers in serious ways—not just today with perhaps a minor injury but down a long, bumpy road into a future where serious health consequences loom. In my mind, preventing that from happening sooner rather than later is even more important than any game. Lucky for me, when we improve their sleep (and their health), their game improves too!

A lot of why we are more successful when we sleep well has to do with what's happening inside our brains when we sleep. Turn to the next chapter for a closer look inside this fascinating yet mysterious "brainwashing" process—and why it's so critical to our present and future health.

PART II:

THE RX FACTOR: SLEEP IS MEDICINE

Chapter 4

The Best Kind of "Brainwashing"

Sleep Vigilanteism: One of the brain's most
powerful sedatives is wakefulness in sunshine.

Back in the early 1990s, when I was a teenager in India (watching *Baywatch*, jamming to Michael Jackson's *Dangerous* album, and learning Guns N' Roses riffs on the guitar so I could impress girls—basically just trying my hardest to be the coolest 13-year-old around), my father attended a management retreat for work. But this wasn't like the other skills-training getaways he'd attended in the past for his job at Indian Railways. This time, when he rolled his suitcase back into our home six weeks later, he'd changed a little bit—and become a big believer in yoga (or "yog"—rhymes with "vogue"—in the original Sanskrit), meditation, and mindfulness. The practices were taught to the managers to help them regulate stress levels, improve concentration and performance, and better interact with their employees.

When you consider that yoga originated in my home country and that it was already an integral part of Indian culture—its roots stretching back thousands of years—perhaps my father's ready acceptance isn't so surprising. But back in the '90s, these ancient beliefs were starting to feel modern again, with global mainstream acceptance building momentum even in places like America and Britain. Of course, it didn't feel very modern to me when I'd see him meditating on the couch in the early afternoon as I ran past on my way to play cricket with my friends.

My sister and I began to notice this new behavior of his every single day. He would come home from work on his lunch break and dedicate 15 minutes of that time to resting on the couch in meditation. (Sometimes he even fell asleep.) He told us not to bother him unless it was an emergency. He got so good at this, in fact, that he could recline in quiet stillness, eyes closed, in the middle of our chaotic household and its racket of ringing phones, chiming doorbells, and the clanging of pots, pans, and dishes being cleared from the table.

He'd elevated these daily "power naps" into something of an art form, and it always kind of fascinated me. Sometimes he'd share how refreshed he felt after. No wonder: These little sleep sessions rested his brain and calmed his mind in important ways—we just didn't fully understand it at the time. And when I was young and feeling invincible, I didn't think I needed to nap. Not me! That all changed a couple of decades later, when I found myself almost crushed by exhaustion on a particularly difficult day in my early 30s at the sleep lab.

I'd been up for 28 hours straight, admitting patients and doing an overnight shift at the hospital—from 8 a.m., all through the day past midnight, until noon the *next* day.

The terrible realization dawned on me that I had to make a three-hour drive to Chicago that evening, but the task felt impossible to my fatigued self. I remembered my father's naps and thought, *Hey, why don't I just go to the sleep lab and rest for a few minutes?* And so I did exactly that. I set my alarm for 20 minutes (otherwise I knew I'd sleep all afternoon) and felt amazing after! Also, the drive to Chicago went just fine.

That's when this realization struck me: Wow! I can use this to my advantage! I'd learned the art of napping from my dad, but by this point, I knew the science too. I'd also hit that season in my life where fatherhood, cascading work commitments, and hectic schedules frequently intersected in sometimes messy ways. I focused on turning the infrequent, random 15-minute nap into an important daily habit for me. (Like father, like son.) These days, I often head up to the sleep lab on the second floor (my office is on the first), throw a blanket over myself, and set the timer on my phone. And when I'm too lazy to trudge up that flight of stairs, I unroll a yoga mat on the floor of my office and take my snooze there. I try my best to stick to this schedule on weekends too. (It's tough, but I do try.)

These small breaks might seem inconsequential, but they energize my thoughts for the afternoon and improve my evenings with my family. And those days when I miss my nap, I can really feel my energy crashing by 3 p.m.—that's when you'll find me downing a sugary coffee and rushing around the sleep clinic in my white coat, eclair doughnut in hand.

The Power of 900 Seconds

Your body goes into a brief, natural lull between the hours of noon and 3 p.m. every day, usually for about 30 to 45 minutes max. Keeping your mind still for 15 minutes (or 900 seconds) during this time holds amazing power. A simple 15-minute "recharge" will make you more

- accurate,
- agile,
- alert,
- emotionally regulated,
- focused, and
- productive.

NASA studied the effects of naps ("controlled rest") on pilots and found that those who took naps "maintained consistent performance."[1] Research has shown that 15 to 20 minutes is the sweet spot; when naps last 45 minutes or even a couple of hours, it's a problem—you're messing up your sleep-wake circadian rhythm or possibly harboring a mood or sleep disorder.

Why Sleep Feels So Good

Whether it's a quick rest in the middle of the day or a long, restful night cozied up under the covers, we all know that quality sleep just feels good. Why is this?

It all comes down to the brain, the focus of this chapter. I'm going to get a little geeky and scientific here, but it's only because I believe that once you understand the vital functions unfolding inside your brain as you sleep, this awareness will encourage you to take your own sleep more seriously. Because sleeping five hours a night just doesn't cut it. Just as we cannot grow a healthy baby by compressing a human pregnancy from nine months to just three, we cannot live our best, healthiest life with fewer than seven or eight hours per night (and sometimes even nine, depending on your personal needs).

Those seven, eight, or nine hours of sleep at night are so vital to your brain. Imagine that sleep is a premium washing machine with a lifetime warranty—but instead of washing dirty clothes, it cleanses the gunk and junk that builds up in your brain all day long. Similar to the cycles of a washing machine, the cycles of sleep

- cleanse, restore, and replenish your brain;
- align, organize, and archive memories, knowledge, and all that you learned that day;
- flush out toxins;
- prepare you physically and mentally for the next day; and
- probably do even more things yet to be discovered.

Recent studies have found that as we sleep, our brain cells shrink a little bit, and the spaces between these neurons increase. And when you're sleeping, the flow of cerebrospinal fluid (CSF) around these neurons speeds up twofold.[2] (CSF is basically the fluid that our brains and spinal cords bathe and float in all our lives.) When CSF flows really fast, it's like your pressure washer. It sprays away the toxins and gunk that have accumulated from a hard day's work. Now imagine that process not happening optimally if you sleep poorly—and the negative health effects sure to result.

Some of that gunk is a metabolic waste product called beta-amyloid. Beta-amyloid is the stuff you *don't* want sticking around in your brain for long. It's the trash that needs to be collected every morning. Researchers have shown in mice and in humans that sleep deprivation leads to more beta-amyloid in the brain in the areas responsible for memory.[3] Scientists, connecting the dots, have since linked beta-amyloid accumulation to dementia and Alzheimer's disease. Not good.

That's what I mean by "brainwashing" (in the most positive sense). We all know how good we feel when we get adequate quality and quantity of sleep. And just as you can't really rush the cycles of your washing machine, you also can't rush sleep. When you remove hours of sleep from your night, you're eliminating important cleansing cycles required for brain function and restoration.

A Peek inside Your Brain during Sleep

You can think of your brain as your body's control center for sleep. Different parts of the brain light up as you pass through different stages of the sleep cycle. Figure 4.1 is an illustration I created a few years ago with one of my students. It shows the different parts of the brain and hormones involved in sleep.

If we could peek inside our brains while we slept, we would see a beautiful symphony. Except instead of brass, percussion, strings, and woodwind instruments, the sleep symphony comprises melatonin, adenosine, and GABA. You've heard of melatonin, but what about the rest?

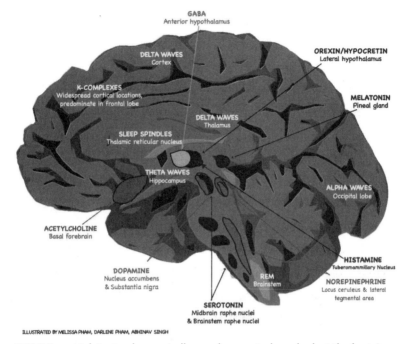

GABA
Anterior hypothalamus

DELTA WAVES
Cortex

OREXIN/HYPOCRETIN
Lateral hypothalamus

K-COMPLEXES
Widespread cortical locations,
predominate in frontal lobe

MELATONIN
Pineal gland

DELTA WAVES
Thalamus

SLEEP SPINDLES
Thalamic reticular nucleus

THETA WAVES
Hippocampus

ALPHA WAVES
Occipital lobe

ACETYLCHOLINE
Basal forebrain

HISTAMINE
Tuberomammillary Nucleus

DOPAMINE
Nucleus accumbens
& Substantia nigra

REM
Brainstem

NOREPINEPHRINE
Locus ceruleus & lateral
tegmental area

SEROTONIN
Midbrain raphe nuclei
& Brainstem raphe nuclei

ILLUSTRATED BY MELISSA PHAM, DARLENE PHAM, ABHINAV SINGH

FIGURE 4.1. Melatonin, sleep spindles, and more: A closer look at the brain's dynamic sleep symphony

First things first. As night falls and the light begins to dim (assuming we've had our 14-plus hours of wakefulness), your body starts to naturally produce melatonin from the pineal gland, which is located in the center of your brain, where the two halves join together. This action influences various other parts of the brain to activate sleep hormone production. Almost every cell in the body has a receptor that responds to this signal, and it's all championed by melatonin.

Along with melatonin, you have adenosine, a chemical that builds up throughout the day as you use energy. Adenosine buildup causes more and more sleep drive (a.k.a. homeostatic sleep drive).

Melatonin plus adenosine triggers the VLPO (ventrolateral preoptic nucleus, a cluster of neurons in the anterior hypothalamus); when this gets stimulated, it releases GABA (gamma-aminobutyric acid), a chemical messenger that inhibits all our wake-promoting centers and promotes non-REM sleep. Epinephrine, dopamine, serotonin—all of these get shut down by GABA. GABA is also what makes us start to feel more and more drowsy and helps us get into states of sleep.

We can also look at this process with a flight analogy. In this case, melatonin is your boarding pass that gets you onto the plane, and adenosine is your seat belt buckling you in for an eight-hour flight. VLPO and GABA are the jet fuel the plane uses to take off. With all the parts working in unison, your sleep engine revs on, and you take to the skies, headed for dreamland.

The Caffeine Conundrum

Who doesn't love a hot cup of joe first thing in the morning—or even in the afternoon? It's the most commonly used legal stimulant in the world. But caffeine has an interesting connection to adenosine worth mentioning.

When you are awake and using energy, your brain burns ATP (adenosine triphosphate). ATP molecules are like little energy packets. After you use them up, there is leftover adenosine, which is kind of like an empty can after you've gulped down everything inside. The more adenosine that builds up through the day (imagine a pile of empty cans on your porch getting taller and wider), the more fatigued and sleepy you are going to feel. When you sleep, all those cans get cleared away. The porch gets cleaned, and you wake up feeling refreshed (until you build up more cans during the day and so on).

When you're feeling tired and you drink caffeine, the adenosine doesn't get cleared away. Caffeine is an artificial adenosine receptor antagonist— meaning it functions more like putting a blanket over the pile of empty cans so you don't have to look at them (but they're still there). So you might feel better for a few hours, but then once the caffeine wears off—in about six hours, it reduces by half—you feel worse. The blanket gets pulled away, and now there are even *more* cans of adenosine. There are so many bottles now, they're rolling around and clanking and making a mess. (Welcome to your caffeine crash.)

People on caffeine are awake, but they're not the sharpest. Your eyes are open, but the brain is not. You're "fake awake," and we've all felt this, haven't we? Nothing refreshes us like sleep—not even caffeine. And now you know why.

If you wake up in the morning and cannot do without your coffee to achieve wakefulness, then that's a signal that all the adenosine trash wasn't cleared away while you slept. It's a subtle hint you're not getting enough sleep, and it's something to pay attention to.

The Stages of Sleep

Your sleep is made up of four stages: stages 1, 2, 3, and REM (rapid eye movement). Technically, there are five stages of sleep, but stage 4 is mostly reserved for research purposes, so for this book, we'll think of stages 3 and 4 as combined into stage 3, as is mostly used in the clinical world.

Stage 1 doesn't last long—you can imagine it's like the short time you spend taxiing down the runway before take-off. You're getting drowsy; you shut your book, turn the lights down, and close your eyes. In stage 1, which makes up about 5 percent of the night, you experience light, non-REM sleep. The plane has just left the ground.

As the plane ascends, passes 10,000 feet, and starts to change direction, you enter deeper states of sleep. We're now in **stage 2**, where you spend the bulk of your night. Your brain waves, predominantly theta waves, start to get a little slower and more synchronized.

In stage 2, sleep spindles make their appearance. These are little non-REM bits or bursts of faster brain wave activity generated from the thalamus area that we can record on brain scans. These bursts only last a few seconds, and we have some theories on their function. We think they are an inhibiting process, working to block light interruptions to sleep. So if your neighbor is knocking on the door at an inopportune time, it's as if your brain is putting earmuffs on so you don't hear it. That's one theory, anyway.

During this stage, we also see K-complexes (brief, large waves that unequivocally mark sleep stage 2 NREM, or non-REM). Their function and origin are felt to be similar to the spindles (mentioned above) that shield the sleeping brain from minor awakening and promote sleep continuity.

Once you enter **stage 3**, the plane is getting closer to its destination, and your brain waves slow *way* down. They turn into delta waves—big, slow, and synchronized. We call this stage "slow wave" sleep or "deep sleep." Your muscles are completely relaxed. Your blood pressure has dropped. Your brain and body temperatures are cooling off, and your breathing becomes slow and regular. This is the stage where muscles are being repaired and memories are being consolidated. "Trash" is being cleared from the brain and body, and growth hormone is released. You're dreaming here, but you won't recall it.

We see bone growth, cellular repair, muscle growth, healing, immunity being strengthened, learning, comprehension, and more all happening at this stage. Your CSF is moving quicker now too, pressure washing all the bad stuff away. This stage of sleep is so, so important. This is the high-quality part you don't want to miss. Every time you cut your sleep short, you miss out on these important functions. And remember, before you can experience stage 3, the bulk of which happens in the first half of your sleep period, you must first pass through stages 1 and 2.

How important is this stage of sleep? A recent study published in *Nature Communications* found that chronically underslept folks between the ages of 50 and 60 who slept fewer than six hours a night had an almost 30 percent higher chance of developing dementia.[4] This is quite stark, and other bodies of research have pointed in the same direction. We don't know for sure if lack of sleep in middle age is the cause, but it's a risk association we shouldn't ignore.

The Paradox of Paradoxical Sleep

Perhaps the most captivating and mysterious sleep stage of all is REM sleep, where dreams and sleep interlace, where the brain scan of a person dreaming looks exactly as if they were awake. (That's the paradox.) When we get our requisite eight hours, we spend around two of those in REM (broken up into three or four smaller pieces that get bigger as the night progresses—the longest of which clocks in at around 40 minutes), predominantly in the second half of sleep.

Why do we dream? And what do dreams mean? Dream states enchant us so much they inspire literature (*Alice in Wonderland*), movies like *Inception* (2010), popular songs, folklore, art, poetry, and even the name of the band R.E.M. (another favorite of mine back in the early 1990s). REM sleep was discovered in 1953 at the University of Chicago; I remember interviewing there and seeing the plaque on the wall commemorating it. Seventy years later, there's still so much we don't know.

When we sink into REM, those giant, slow delta waves change. Suddenly they get shorter, smaller, and faster and last for 20 to 30 minutes. Our bodies slip into a temporary paralyzed state with zero muscle tone, coupled with intriguing darting eye movements, from which we derived the term *REM*. We use almost as much energy when dreaming during REM sleep as we do when we're awake. Our body temperature falls to its lowest during REM sleep around two-thirds of the way into the sleep flight; paradoxically, our pulse rate goes haywire and gets more erratic; our brains consume as much oxygen and glucose as when we're awake.

We can often remember our REM dreams upon waking, though they tend to dissipate after that. Recent data have led scientists to believe our dreams are associated with creative endeavors and mental health, including dealing with positive and negative emotions and memories.[5] We also now know that people deprived of REM have shorter life-spans.[6]

You can research dream meanings and symbols online or in books or meet with an "expert" dream interpreter, but the explanations are less scientific and more subjective in my opinion. We've all woken up from dreams that have left unanswered questions in our minds. Maybe dreams reveal important spiritual meanings, or maybe they're just insignificant electrical impulses. For this book, we'll table that topic and move instead into another brain-related sleep subject that fascinates me just as much: parasomnias.

When Sleep Throws a Curve Ball

Sometimes things go awry while you are sleeping, or during that fine line between drifting to sleep or waking up. These events are called **parasomnias**. Back in the 1930s, Henri Roger, a French researcher, reportedly coined the term *parasomnie* by combining *para* (Greek for "alongside of") with *somnus* (Latin for "sleep"). The term stuck, and we still use it today.

Examples of abnormal behaviors characteristic of parasomnias include sleepwalking, sleep terrors, sleep talking, sleep paralysis, sleep-related eating disorders, nightmares, and REM behavior disorder. Some happen during REM sleep; others occur strictly during non-REM sleep. Parasomnias can be frightening for the patient (and often their spouse), but even worse, sometimes they signal a serious, undiagnosed brain disorder.

I once had a patient named Luis who came to me after suffering from strange episodes in his sleep. This guy was healthy, a baseball coach in his 50s. But Luis was acting out baseball games in his dreams—swinging the bat, pitching the ball, and announcing the game as if it were a real, live event in the stadium. And in his sleep, he'd thrash around the bed and accidentally land on his wife or hit her. He sometimes knocked the lamp and everything else off the nightstand. He once flew off the bed with so much force that he injured his knee. He was also exhausted during the day, for acting out these dreams was consuming a ton of energy. Bedtime had become a dangerous event—so bad, in fact, that his wife now slept in another room.

Was he taking drugs? Did he have a brain tumor? Was he going to have a seizure? His primary care doctor had questions and sent him to me for answers, as these events occurred exclusively during his sleep period.

I suspected a parasomnia of the REM type, which was soon confirmed by a sleep study in our lab. Traditionally, during REM sleep, all your muscles are paralyzed. So you can dream you are jumping, but you don't actually jump. It's kind of like using the parking brake on a steep street in San Francisco. If you engage this brake after you park, your car isn't going to roll down the hill out of control. Your body should also have a "parking brake" for certain muscles that engages during REM sleep and keeps you safe. We all have bizarre dreams, but no one gets hurt, right?

But with Luis, something was wrong with his parking brake. While in REM, my team witnessed his hand and leg muscles twitching. He mumbled a lot. He didn't "act out" the way he did at home, but we got the confirmation we needed that the normal muscle paralysis you expect to see during dreaming just wasn't happening. His body's parking brake was not engaged.

We use medications to treat REM behavior disorder, and so we started him on a low dose of Clonazepam, also known as Klonopin, which is commonly used to treat anxiety disorders. In just half a week, his episodes reduced dramatically. We upped the dose a tiny bit after that, and they disappeared completely. His sleep improved so much that his wife could sleep in the room again. Another success story, right?

Not so fast. We improved his sleep, yes. But sleep physicians such as myself also know that REM behavior disorder is a strong prediagnostic symptom of Parkinson's disease. This is actually how actor Alan Alda discovered he had Parkinson's. In 2018, he shared with *CBS This Morning* that in a dream, he acted out throwing a "sack of potatoes" at his attacker, except that what he actually did was throw a pillow at his wife. This experience, in addition to reading an article about these kinds of dreams and their connection to Parkinson's, led him to ask his doctor for a scan, which ultimately led to his diagnosis.

As for my patient Luis, I followed up with him year after year, and he continued to take a low dose of Klonopin and sleep peacefully. Klonopin, a Valium derivative, is known for being habit forming, but we use such a small dose to treat parasomnias that we typically don't see a tolerance develop or a need for escalating dosages.

Seven years later, at his annual appointment, I learned that indeed Luis had begun to exhibit features of Parkinson's. I had hoped this would not happen, but the link between REM behavior disorder and Parkinson's is hard to ignore. According to one 2015 study, 30 percent of people with this specific parasomnia go on to develop Parkinson's, dementia, or a similar neurodegenerative disorder within three years. The figure rises to 66 percent within seven and a half years.[7]

Sleepy versus Tired (Yes, There's a Difference)

People often use the terms *sleepy* and *tired* interchangeably. But sleep nerds like me know they are not the same thing.

Tired: lack of energy, exhausted, and drained; doesn't relent even after you sleep

Sleepy: feeling drowsy; yawning a lot; feeling an urge to sleep

Just as hunger and thirst are different, so are *sleepy* and *tired*. They can run together but are distinct. For thirst, you need water; for hunger, you need food. For tiredness, you need energy; for sleepiness, you need sleep.

There are a lot of reasons why you may be tired: stress, not eating properly, having a thyroid condition, medication side effects, overexerting yourself. But being sleepy is simpler: You just need sleep. I often find that you can distill or separate the two by sleeping appropriately and then seeing what's left over. Maybe a lot can be improved in your life just by attending to your sleepiness.

On this side of the pond, where siestas are often looked down upon, I see people hiding behind the mask of tiredness when really they're just sleepy. Being tired is a badge of honor: "Wow, no wonder she's tired—she works 80-hour weeks." But being sleepy? "Look at that guy—he's a slacker." We jump to conclusions about people. I'm ready for a sleep revolution in our culture where we *all* welcome sleep and pay attention to it, when it isn't just a passing fad like the novelty of a nap pod in Silicon Valley. Humanity will benefit when we collectively come to value eight hours a night and embrace a short recharge in the day.

Interestingly, I see this a lot with kids, who have sleep needs that exceed ours. I'd say about one-third of kids diagnosed with attention deficit hyperactivity disorder (ADHD) may well have in large part chronic sleep deprivation or a hidden sleep disorder. The meds help them feel better because, in many cases, the stimulant medication has treated their sleepiness. Note that the sleep disorder may not have been addressed yet. And so with these kids, when you treat their sleep deprivation or sleep disorder instead, a lot of those other behavioral problems will resolve.

So ask yourself today, Am I tired or am I just sleepy? (Or am I both?)

Primary versus Secondary Parasomnias

In Luis's case, his REM behavior disorder was the sole sleep disorder present. But sometimes, REM behavior disorder can crop up in addition to something else. In this case, we call it a secondary parasomnia, and we approach the treatment of it differently too.

When I first met my patient Tarek, his was a fascinating case. I will never forget that when he came in to see me, he scored 24/24 on the Epworth Sleepiness Scale. That's almost unheard of! For those who aren't familiar, it's literally the worst score you can get. In the questionnaire, we ask patients to rate from 0 to 3 how likely they are to fall asleep in different scenarios during the day—like reading a book, watching TV, or sitting quietly at their desks after lunch. Tarek was so tired and sleepy, he rated all eight questions as a 3. The man was exhausted and supremely sleepy!

Here was a guy in his early 50s with severe obstructive sleep apnea who could no longer tolerate his CPAP therapy at night. He'd let four years slip by, not using it, and ended up in my office feeling excessively sleepy, dangerously drowsy, and absolutely miserable. He used to fall asleep during our appointments, and his wife would speak for him—that's how sleepy he was!

But as if his sleep apnea wasn't bad enough, he had begun to experience excessive dream reenactments over the years, and they were worsening. He'd talk loudly at night, fall out of bed, and wake up at least three times a night. Once in his sleep, he punched the drywall above his headboard and dented it. Another time, he fell out of bed, hit his head on the nightstand, and had to get stitches. His wife told me he'd pushed the bed against the wall on one side in order to feel a little safer.

Tarek suffered from terrible sleep apnea plus fragmentation from his parasomnia. I wondered, Which was the primary problem? I wanted some fresh data.

We put him through a sleep study, and the results astounded me. His sleep apnea was so severe that he suffered 99 breathing pauses per hour. (Normal is 5; severe is 30.) He also presented abnormal limb movements consistent with REM behavior disorder. We sent him home with instructions to use his CPAP, but he still couldn't find success with it. He simply wasn't able to use it.

I had to do something. My thinking was that his parasomnia was likely a secondary problem caused by the sleep apnea. If we could treat the sleep apnea, perhaps the parasomnia would go away. He would have to find a way to use the dreaded CPAP machine.

And so for Tarek, the approach I chose wasn't meds; it was a behavioral therapy called desensitization, which is commonly deployed to address various phobias. Desensitization means that if a person is scared of spiders, you conquer their fear by getting them used to looking at pictures of spiders, taking them to a spider farm, and ultimately holding a spider in their hand. For Tarek, the CPAP machine was his spider.

He'd developed a powerful aversion, so I suggested that we reintroduce him—slowly—to his CPAP machine again. When the case is this severe, it requires lots of patience for both the practitioner and the patient. In the beginning, I just wanted him to look at the machine for a few minutes a day. He didn't have to touch it or wear it; he just had to look at it. When he conquered that step, I had him hold the CPAP in his hand for a few minutes a day. He didn't have to put it on. I just wanted him to get used to the feeling of it and not fear it so much.

When enough time passed that he finally felt ready, I had him touch it to his face a few times a day. Eventually, we moved to him wearing it for a short nap, slowly breaking him in with pressure. I did ask him to trim his beard at this point, because when you have a lot of facial hair, you're going to get a lot of leakage. He trimmed his beard, and in time we got him tolerating his CPAP . . . slowly, slowly. We made small adjustments to the pressure and exhale relief settings to get it just right.

It was a miracle moment when, four months after his initial sleep study, Tarek came back to see me. He was wearing his CPAP at night, and he'd dropped from 24 down to 13 on the Epworth Sleepiness Scale. (Less than 10 is considered normal.) He was sleeping a whole lot better, his parasomnia activity improved, they got the drywall repaired, and he even stayed awake during our appointment! His blood pressure got better too, his mood improved, and he was able to lower the antianxiety meds from his psychiatrist.

Just Breathe . . .

A CPAP interface is like a new pair of shoes. They don't feel exactly comfortable straight out of the box, do they? You have to break them in first. Or imagine sticking your head out of a car window traveling at 40 miles per hour. The air is coming at your face pretty hard, isn't it? With a CPAP, you just need to be calm, breathe slowly with the machine, and not get panicked by the air that's coming. Most of my patients have found that a little vitamin P (patience) is all they need to get used to it.

The last time I saw Tarek, in 2021, he was doing great. His breathing pauses at night had dropped from 99 per night to less than 15. We consider this a success! It's not perfect, but the man loves his beard. He'd decided to grow it back even if that meant the CPAP would leak a little. We don't chase perfection here, and I can make peace with that. The important takeaway is we improved his life.

I will continue to monitor Tarek's sleep and watch for signs of Parkinson's. But because his REM behavior disorder was likely a secondary and not primary parasomnia, I'm not quite as concerned as I was with Luis. The science is still evolving, but my hope is that he does not go on to develop Parkinson's.

Parasomnias

Non-REM

- sleepwalking
- sleep terrors (or night terrors): most common in children ages 4–12
- sleep-related eating disorders
- teeth grinding (bruxism)

REM

- nightmares
- sleep paralysis
- REM behavior disorder

A New Paradigm: Then versus Now

Our beliefs on sleep have changed so much since the 20th century. Back then, everyone thought sleep was a complete shutdown. The old-fashioned belief was that everything in your brain and body locked up, closed down, and rested for the night.

We know better now. Now we know that more than 25 percent of our nighttime brain-wave activity is very high. This is not just due to dream sleep but also the result of our CSF racing through and cleaning our brain cells up to two times faster than during normal waking hours. Our sleep is that precious time when our body cleans, restores, repairs, and rejuvenates. It's a harmonious routine of slow and fast activities aimed to repair: Growth hormone is triggered. Your immune system is strengthened. Your blood sugar balances—insulin is being suppressed so you don't get hungry at night. The antidiuretic hormone is released so you don't have to use the bathroom frequently at night. All of these processes (and more) synchronize at night so your body can focus on much-needed repair. This maintenance program is so essential, in fact, that your body will prioritize it for your entire life.

But do most of us think about this when we think of "health"? Not really. The World Health Organization (WHO) defines health as not just the absence of disease but also the embodiment of well-being: physical, mental, and social. This is a good definition, but it does not go far enough. I urge them to add "sleep health" to their definition of health. Optimal sleep makes us happy, after all. (This idea is so important, I've devoted the next chapter to it.)

Just because your eyes are shut does not mean you are sleeping well or attaining your highest state of well-being. Also, hyperfocusing on nutrition and exercise alone to achieve optimal health is not sufficient—high-quality sleep must also factor into the equation every single day (and night). But before you can evaluate or fix something, you need to know to look at it. I hope this book helps encourage readers with this step.

The field of sleep medicine continues to ascend in importance, especially now with the American Academy of Sleep Medicine's political action committee (PAC) working to promote awareness of sleep disorders, funding in sleep science research, and legislation supporting sleep as it relates to public health. It's exciting to think about where the next century will take us. How long will it take us all to wake up to the importance of sleep? Will this be the "eureka" of modern health sciences?

Chapter 5

50 Ways Sleep Makes You Happy

*Sleep Vigilanteism: Sleep is a carafe filled
with free, zero-calorie, all-natural happy
juice. How much would you like?*

Nobody ever says they feel *worse* after getting an optimal night of sleep. It's like drinking fresh water or taking in the beauty of a vivid sunset. But instead of seeking out the happiness it brings, so many of us continue to take sleep for granted—night after night, year after year.

Scientists have aimed to study sleep and happiness by quantifying life satisfaction levels. And they've found (surprise!) that happier people sleep better. But there are limits to such surveys. Do people define happiness the same way? Do happier people get better sleep because they are already happy? Or are they happy because they slept better?

At this point in my life, after being fortunate enough to help more than 7,000 patients sleep much better and also experiencing the benefits of sleep firsthand, maybe we don't need to sort out this chicken-and-egg scenario. I say you can

have both. You can have the chicken *and* the egg: Sleep makes
you happy, and happiness makes you sleep!

It felt really good to compile the following list for you.
It's almost overwhelming to see how many bountiful gifts
sleep gives us all in one place. And because the opposite of
happy is unhappy (just as the opposite of "somnia" is insomnia), I conclude the chapter with some important information about insomnia, a disorder that often surfaces following
stressful life events and when we are at our lowest.

With that said, here are 50 (yes, 50!) powerful ways sleep
makes you happy:

Sleep Helps You Cultivate a Happy Body

1. **More energy:** As you learned in chapter 4, when you get
   the optimal quality and quantity of sleep, your body repairs
   and clears away the metabolic waste products that accumulate in your brain as you use energy. Eight hours of sleep
   "power washes" all the gunk away and rests your body so you
   can step out of bed feeling refreshed, restored, and revitalized. It recharges your battery so you can power through the
   day—whether that means staying alert in meetings or helping
   your kids with their homework after a long day of work (like
   my strong-willed 10-year-old).

2. **Slower aging:** A 2015 study by UCLA researchers found
   that just a single night of sleep loss was linked to DNA damage and biological aging in adults.[1] And in another UCLA
   study from 2021 that looked at new moms six months
   after childbirth, those who slept less than seven hours a
   night aged three to seven years faster than their well-rested
   counterparts.[2]

3. **A higher pain tolerance:** It is well documented that "sleep loss amplifies the experience of pain," as a 2019 study published in the *Journal of Neuroscience* noted.[3] Another study in 2015 found that insomnia sufferers had a lower tolerance for pain than those who slept well.[4] Studies have also shown that fragmented sleep is associated with increased pain in people with fibromyalgia.[5] Like so many systems affected by sleep, it's an inverse relationship: More pain means less sleep. It's a vicious cycle too: sleep loss = pain = sleep loss . . .

4. **Fewer medications:** I've seen this time and again with my very own patients! When we are able to restore their sleep, oftentimes they go on to drop their sleeping pills, reduce antidepressants, and sometimes even lower their heart or blood pressure medications.

5. **Fewer headaches:** All of us dislike headaches, whether they're uncomfortable tension headaches or debilitating migraines. Science has shown that sleep problems like insomnia can trigger headaches, and a 2021 study published in the journal *Neurology* found that those who got migraines also logged less REM sleep.[6] In addition, as noted by the International Classification of Headache Disorders (ICHD-3), the common sleep disorder obstructive sleep apnea (which often goes undiagnosed) can easily add to headaches, especially morning headaches.

6. **Less risk of diabetes:** Sleep loss seems to put otherwise healthy individuals at a higher risk of developing diabetes. Research has indicated that even one night of sleep deprivation can induce insulin resistance in the body.[7] That's not so sweet, is it?

7. **Reduced back pain:** Back pain can interfere with an optimal night's rest, but sleeping poorly can also make your back hurt

more. Protecting your sleep every day (and going through *all* the sleep cycles I talked about in chapter 4) will give your body its best chance at resting and healing that sore back. Make sure your pillow and mattress are comfortable and supportive too.

8. **Healthy hair:** Different hormones, such as the human growth hormone, affect hair growth. Early research suggests that melatonin may play a role as well. Sleeping well keeps hormones like these in balance; meanwhile, sleep apnea has been associated with male pattern baldness and thinning hair. Lack of sleep also causes stress, which can lead to graying hair and hair loss.

9. **Muscle repair:** Marathon runners already know this, but getting those crucial eight-plus hours of shut-eye every night is essential to muscle repair. Research has shown that high-quality sleep helps heal sore or injured muscles during the deeper sleep states.[8] If you regularly chop off the last two hours of your sleep, you're missing out on the full restorative benefits of sleep.

10. **A stronger heart:** Your heart is a muscle too, so take extra good care of it with adequate sleep. Lack of sleep is associated with a whole host of heart problems, including hypertension, heart failure, arrhythmia, and atherosclerosis (plaque buildup in the arteries, which causes poor circulation). A 2019 study found a 20 percent increase in heart attacks in people who slept less than six hours a night.[9] People already suffering from cardiovascular problems must especially prioritize protecting their hearts—which means protecting their sleep too. Perhaps not surprisingly, significantly more heart attacks occur on the Monday following the start of spring Daylight Saving Time, when we all have to get up an hour earlier. Additionally, more heart attacks have been seen between the hours of midnight and 6 a.m. in folks with untreated sleep apnea.[10]

OBESITY AND SLEEP LOSS: A *WEIGH* BIGGER PROBLEM THAN YOU THINK

Obesity is not an easy problem to solve, but the connection of appetite to sleep dysregulation should not be ignored. The science shows us that sleep loss makes you hungrier and less disciplined. When you're tired, you're not reaching for a kale salad—you want calorie-dense comfort foods like doughnuts, fries, and candy bars.

But how does this translate to the real world? Does healthy sleep *really* make that much of a difference in your waistline?

The answer is a solid yes. After several studies pointing in favor of this argument over the last decade, a recent study in February 2022 from the University of Chicago and the University of Wisconsin–Madison found that participants who extended their sleep by 1.2 hours per night (with the goal of 8.5 hours in bed) reduced their caloric intake by 270 calories per day. That adds up to about 26 pounds of weight lost over three years, assuming the healthy sleep habit is maintained.[11]

The takeaway? If losing weight is a priority for you, you must make healthy sleep of the right quantity and quality an integral part of your weight-loss plan. As the saying goes, "You snooze, you lose"—but in this case, the cool thing is that you're losing weight!

11. **Less weight gain:** When you deprive your body of sleep, you crave more food and snacks to find enough energy to get through the day. You can thank ghrelin for that; the levels of this hormone increase when sleep is lost. Ghrelin makes you feel hungry—the very name of it sounds like a "growling" stomach! In addition, when you're fatigued, you also lack the willpower and energy to exercise. What does less exercise plus that daily 3 p.m. doughnut get you? Unwanted pounds. Studies have also shown that the risk of obesity increases in those who sleep less than five hours per night—and obesity increases your cancer risk (see #19). Sleep is an important secret to maintaining a healthy weight.[12]

12. **Fewer asthma attacks:** A 2020 study found that adults with asthma who slept too little (five hours or less a night) or too much (more than nine hours a night) were more likely to have had an asthma attack or an overnight hospital stay in the past year.[13] It's worth noting that the need to sleep nine or more hours per night may be a sign of an underlying illness or sleep disorder.

13. **Improved athletic performance:** Whether you like to spend your weekends golfing, swimming, mountain biking, or shooting hoops on the basketball court, proper sleep brings out your best. As you learned in chapter 3, athletes who sleep more see a significant improvement in their performance. A 2011 Stanford study found that basketball players who slept 10 hours per night increased their accuracy in free throws by 9 percent in addition to faster sprint times.[14] The good news is you don't have to be a professional athlete to experience the physical benefits of sleep.

14. **Sharper reflexes:** When people are sleep deprived for even one day, their reaction times lag and their reflexes slow. This can take a toll on both you and our society as a whole as we power through our days, making tough decisions, crossing paths with others, and sometimes even operating danger-ous machinery. (Just think back to all those accidents I talked about in chapter 2, "The Hidden Truths of Sleep Loss.") To ensure your reflexes are at their best, you simply cannot neglect your sleep.

15. **Improved balance:** When you're sleep deprived, you're just as impaired as if you were drunk. You're more likely to sway and lose postural stability and less likely to catch yourself if you trip or fall. When older adults sleep poorly and wake up off-balance, they are more likely to suffer from dangerous and even life-threatening falls and potential fractures.

16. **Less prone to injuries:** Sleep protects you from more than just falls. When you lose sleep, you're more likely to get injured in general (see #14 and #15)—whether it happens on the sports field or in a workplace accident. Sleep is so import-ant that a 20-year Swedish study published in 2002 found that workers suffering from sleep problems were twice as likely to die in workplace-related accidents.[15]

17. **A stronger immune system:** Sleep sharpens your defenses. Research has shown that when we sleep seven-plus hours a night, our immune system gets stronger by producing the ingredients T cells need (like integrin) to identify, target, and fight off infection.[16] But when we lose sleep, this functionality weakens. An impaired immune system leaves you vulnerable to a wide variety of diseases and infections—but when you invest in the best sleep

possible, you reap the rewards of robust immunity, which is especially important during the COVID-19 pandemic. (For more on the pandemic and its connection to sleep, turn to chapter 8.)

18. **More effective vaccines:** Since we're on the subject of immunity, vaccines have been shown to be more effective in individuals who get regular, adequate sleep. A 2020 study published in the *International Journal of Behavioral Medicine* found that "shorter sleep duration . . . was associated with fewer antibodies" following the flu vaccine.[17] With the coronavirus still spreading around the globe, getting adequate sleep before and after your vaccination is going to be a crucial component of your immune response.

19. **Less risk of cancer:** Although causal relationships have not been established yet, mounting research is beginning to associate increased cancer risk with night shift work. (Night shift workers tend to experience sleep imbalances.)[18] And in another preprint journal review (as of press time), study participants with obstructive sleep apnea and hypoxemia (lower oxygenation of the blood due to breathing pauses at night) showed an elevated cancer risk.[19]

Genes experience crucial repair while we sleep, and we know that sleeping poorly correlates with DNA damage. Preliminary small-scale research shows that melatonin, which is believed to be a tumor disruptor and DNA protector, also gets suppressed when you deprive yourself of sleep.[20] Even though the mechanisms may not be fully understood, respecting your sleep is one thing you can do to lower your risk of cancer.

Sleep Supports a Happy Sense of Self

20. **Better emotional regulation:** Losing control of emotions happens to all of us sometimes, but those who sleep well are less triggered and better able to stay in control. It's an emotional superpower even backed up by science: A 2015 study published in the *Journal of Neuroscience* found that sleep-deprived subjects who logged lower amounts of REM sleep showed "a profound decline in cognitive control of emotion."[21] And a 2021 study published in *Behavioral Sleep Medicine* found that subjects who missed out on REM sleep were more likely to react aversively to photos of negative images.[22] You'll be in a better state to resolve, rationalize, and put away the bad experiences of your life, such as an argument with your boss, if you cherish your nightly sleep. Remember when you were little and you had a bad day, your grandma would say, "Just sleep on it"? It's so true!

21. **More emotional resilience:** The term *emotional resilience* refers to your ability to react to unexpected stressful situations and cope with the ups and downs of life. When you lose sleep, you're in a terrible mood, your thoughts become more negative, you feel more isolated than normal, you're triggered by the smallest thing, and you have a harder time remembering important information that can help you problem-solve effectively. All of these factors and more impact your emotional resilience. The more regular sleep you can get, the healthier and stronger (emotionally) you will feel.

22. **A positive outlook on life:** Are you a glass-half-full or glass-half-empty kind of person? It may depend on your sleeping pattern. A 2019 study from the University of Illinois

at Urbana-Champaign—which surveyed participants twice, five years apart—found that optimists tended to sleep longer (six to nine hours per night) and experience higher-quality sleep compared to pessimists.[23] Their carafe of OJ is filled with "optimism juice."

23. **Lower risk of depression:** When you think about sleep and how it affects our mental health and emotional state, perhaps it's not so surprising that research shows that people who chronically sleep less are more likely to suffer from depression. People who sleep poorly also have a harder time pushing through the winter blues. Depression can certainly cause sleep disorders, but insomnia is also widely considered to be a risk factor for developing depression.[24] (Don't miss my section on "The Insomnia Connection," which follows this list.) Mental health is so important because these kinds of problems lead to other worse problems; they don't happen in a silo. Mood disorders and sleep disorders are good friends; they generally follow each other around.

24. **Less anxiety:** The amount of REM sleep you get can also affect your anxiety levels. Research from UC Berkeley has shown that even one sleepless night can boost anxiety levels by nearly 30 percent.[25] Not only are you more likely to feel anxious if you lose sleep, but anxiety disorders are also associated with serious sleeping problems, including insomnia and frequent nightmares.

25. **More attractive:** Ever looked in the mirror after a 14-hour flight? Now imagine being sleep deprived for months on end. This book has already shown you in a big way how important sleep is to your body—cognitively, emotionally, and physically. There is truth behind the old adage of "beauty sleep."

Among other things, sleep helps repair cells, lowers inflammation, improves circulation, and helps the body release human growth hormone—all good things. Conversely, lack of sleep may accelerate the aging process, which means more wrinkles, limp hair, puffy eyes, dark circles, and worse. No matter your life stage or age, sleep will help you look like the best, most attractive, rested, and glowing version of yourself. Optimal sleep truly is beauty sleep!

26. **More easily learn new things:** Whether it's a new language, a new piece of music, or a golf swing, sleep—and especially dreaming—helps your brain synthesize and retain new information. According to SleepFoundation.org, getting insufficient sleep can lower your ability to learn new information by 40 percent.[26] It just feels good when your hard work pays off and you can shine, whether you're on the links or strumming a complex arrangement on the guitar.

    Back in the late 1990s, closing in on Y2K while I was in med school, I was learning to play the intro melody bars to "Don't Cry" by Guns N' Roses. Night after night, I would fall asleep practicing it in the dark while on winter break. Guess what? I learned it quickly, and to this day it remains a tune I love to play for my 10-year-old.

27. **Better embody the best version of yourself:** If you sleep poorly all the time, you'll always be that crabby, angry person. Who wants that? But sleep well, and you'll find it easier to show up to life as your best self: fresh, patient, sharp, relaxed, and brimming with optimism.

Healthy Sleep Means Happier Days and Nights

28. **Happier upon waking:** After eight full hours of restful sleep, do you need to hit the snooze button five times? Do you feel exhausted even though the day is just beginning? Do you drag your slippered feet down the hall to the coffeemaker because you can't imagine functioning a single minute without it? No, no, no. We all know how *good* it feels to sleep great. But you have to commit to a full night's rest and protect your sleep every night of your life to get the payoff. Trust me, the payoff is rapid and more instant than you think.

29. **Easier mornings:** Which morning goes more smoothly and is less rushed? The one after you got four hours of sleep, or the one where you luxuriated in eight? Exactly. Optimal sleep sets your whole day up to be a good one. Challenges will still cross your path, and no amount of sleep will ever prevent those completely, but at least you will have more reserves to deal with whatever comes your way.

30. **Safer driving:** A car accident—or even a close escape—is a great way to ruin an otherwise happy day. When you get all your sleep, your reflexes and focus are on point. But things start to deteriorate—fast—when you accumulate sleep loss. It is well established that driving while fatigued and sleepy increases your risk of an accident. And if you drive when you're extremely fatigued and sleepy, that accident could be deadly. (For more on this, turn back to chapter 2, where I discussed the four Ds of dangerous driving.)

31. **Higher career satisfaction:** Let's face it: A big part of feeling happy in your daily life is enjoying your job. Well, sleep helps with that too. A 2015 study from Stockholm University found that employees who slept poorly perceived their work

in a more negative light, were stressed out more, and felt overwhelmed by their workload.[27] It is also well known that poor sleep impairs cognitive performance, so if you want to impress your boss, consider healthy sleep as important as that critical deadline you sweat through lunch to meet.

32. **More money:** What if investing in your sleep could make your bank account a little happier? It's an interesting association you shouldn't ignore. Researchers calculated that deepening sleep by one hour a night increased wages by nearly 5 percent long term according to a 2015 study from UC San Diego.[28] In another study, the CDC found that rich people sleep more than those living below the poverty line.[29]

33. **Less absenteeism:** Sleeping better means a stronger immune system, which means you're better able to fight off headaches and colds and other illnesses. The benefit to your workday is that you're less likely to have to call in sick, which can negatively affect your productivity and stress levels when it happens. A 2017 study from the Sleep Health Foundation uncovered similar findings: Those with sleep problems like insomnia were more likely to take sick days.[30]

    Similarly, another term becoming popular that's also serious but harder to measure is *presenteeism*, which means being present but not at your best. Also attributable to poor sleep, presenteeism can also cost the company more.

34. **Stronger leadership skills:** The physical, emotional, and cognitive benefits that come from regularly sleeping that crucial seven- or eight-plus hours a night means you can shine as a leader—whether that means of your household, in the classroom, on the field, in the boardroom, or elsewhere.

35. **Fewer errors:** Studies have shown that people make more errors when they're sleep deprived, and you are no different. Your days will run more smoothly when you aren't forgetting important details or struggling to pay attention during tasks.

36. **Less jet lag:** Jet lag is never fun—but sleep physicians like me know that if you start out sleep deprived, your jet lag from zipping across time zones will be even *more* painful. It takes days to fully acclimate, but you'll get there sooner if you eliminate your sleep debt ahead of time. I still remember missing my fresh croissant in Paris. The breakfast closed at 10 a.m., and I just couldn't get up in time due to poor preparation for combatting my jet lag.

37. **Better sleep:** When you sleep better . . . you just sleep better. Remember this: Great sleep begets more great sleep! And a poor sleep pattern begets a poorer sleep pattern. If you want to sleep well tomorrow night, sleep well tonight. And then repeat that sequence. When you achieve your optimum sleep every night, you set yourself up for a great day tomorrow—and all the tomorrows after that.

Sleep Helps You Build Happier Relationships

38. **More sociable:** Science has shown that lack of sleep tends to close you off from the world. One Swedish study from 2017 found that photos of sleep-deprived participants were ranked as less approachable and less attractive by strangers compared to photos taken of them after a proper night's rest.[31] And a 2018 UC Berkeley study uncovered evidence that losing sleep makes people less sociable in general, which can increase feelings of loneliness and rejection.[32]

39. **Healthier communication:** When you get your full night's rest, you're less reactive, less aggressive and angry, less frustrated, and more patient. You're more emotionally centered, as explained in #20. The benefit? You're more likely to communicate in a healthy manner with friends, family, and colleagues—and even the DMV attendant who kept you standing in line for 45 minutes even though you had an appointment.

40. **More empathy:** Empathy is a key building block in social relationships—it's the ability (and desire) to relate to people, understand others' feelings, and respond appropriately. Now imagine hindering that ability. Unfortunately, that's exactly what sleep deprivation does: Numerous studies have shown that your capacity for emotional empathy is negatively impacted by sleep loss, a harsh consequence that dismantles your ability to connect with others.

41. **Stronger friendships:** When you're feeling open and empathetic to the world around you, of course those attitudes will spill over into your relationships and strengthen your ability to make and keep friends. Conversely, the emotional impacts of sleep loss *will* negatively impact your relationships. Exhausted, bickering couples can probably relate to this.

42. **More and better sex:** Here's another happy benefit of restful sleep: It ramps up your sex drive and arousal—leading to more and better sex! Lack of sleep, meanwhile, negatively affects libido, a contributing factor to married couples with kids often losing interest in sex. Studies have also shown that sleep deprivation correlates to low testosterone in men, leading to erectile dysfunction and unsatisfactory sexual experiences.[33] Next time you and your partner want to binge-watch your favorite series way past midnight, remember this: Quality sleep = great sex!

HEALTHY SLEEP: AN UNDERVALUED (AND POTENT) APHRODISIAC

One of my patients, a busy piano teacher with four rambunctious children, came to me complaining of depression, exhaustion, snoring, and a low libido. A victim of "sleep divorce," he hadn't slept in the bedroom with his wife for months. He blamed it all on being a workaholic and the stress of parenting, but I suspected otherwise.

Sure enough, a sleep study revealed 93 breathing pauses per hour—a severe case of sleep apnea. After fitting him with a CPAP (and persuading him it would help with many aspects of his health, not just the snoring), he came back to see me in a few months. He'd lost weight, felt great, and had been able to ditch his antidepressants. Even better, although his undiagnosed sleep apnea had left his performance in the bedroom a little flat, since starting treatment, his happy wife assured him his grand upright was hitting all the right notes again.

43. **A better marriage:** When you invest in proper sleep every single night, you're better at resolving conflicts in a healthy manner. You are more patient with your partner. You're more active together and more likely to meet fitness and weight-loss goals together. You're empathetic to each other's feelings, needs, and concerns. And you're having more sex too! You will never see it the other way around: A chronically

sleep-deprived couple is never going to be the happiest couple in the room. Practicing good sleep habits together now will help you build a strong and healthy marriage that can (hopefully) last a lifetime.

Sleep Makes Your Brain Happy

44. **Mentally sharper:** Have you ever struggled to solve a problem only for the solution to pop into your brain after an optimal night's rest? Several studies suggest that full, restful sleep—involving both REM and non-REM sleep—does indeed improve memory, retention, learning, problem-solving, and mental sharpness. This can help you get an edge at work, but even kids benefit from this: Children who sleep well do better academically than those who sleep poorly.

45. **More focused:** You know this firsthand from your own life, and I've seen it in my patients too: Studies show that we're cognitively at our best when we sleep well. You're better able to focus, concentrate, and be more productive when your eyelids don't feel like they have weights on them.

46. **More willpower:** No one said self-improvement was easy. Just think about January 1 and "resolution-itis," when all the well-intentioned people every single year let go of their resolutions after weeks, days, and sometimes just hours. If this sounds familiar, sleep could be the missing piece to your motivational mental blocks. A 2015 study published in *Frontiers in Human Neuroscience* found that sleep-deprived subjects were less able to control impulses and more likely to make poor decisions.[34] So if you haven't slept well, for example, you're setting yourself up to fail when it comes to sticking to your exercise plan (choosing social media scrolling over

going to the gym), reaching your weight-loss goals (grabbing the bag of potato chips instead of blending a pineapple smoothie), and so on. Ironically, if sleeping better is going to be a new priority for you, the only way to get there will be by . . . sleeping better. Sleep is a great way to power up your willpower!

47. **More creative:** I've had many patients who work in the creative fields, from artists to musicians, who come to me not only because they feel miserable from sleeping poorly but also because their creativity suffers. Several studies suggest that full, restful sleep—involving both REM and non-REM stages—does indeed support creative thinking and problem-solving, as I mentioned in #44. It just makes sense that it's harder to be innovative when you're exhausted, when you feel terrible and can't focus, when you're fighting with your spouse, if you have a headache, and so on. Slowly but surely, sleep debt harms our bodies, and we simply don't do our best work when we overextend ourselves. Of course, it can be hard to "turn off" your mind when you're a creative type, and many a tortured artist has suffered from insomnia.

Sleep Is Your Foundation for a Happy Future

48. **Lower health care costs:** When you sleep poorly, you're more likely to get sick, miss work, and go to the doctor. That all costs money—$94.9 billion each year according to one 2021 study that looked at the impacts of sleep disorders on health care utilization.[35] Long-term investment in quality sleep also works in your favor to lower your risk of developing diseases like diabetes or cancer—all of which are very

expensive both financially and in terms of your quality of life. Sleep great now to get your handsome payoff of better health and a better life.

49. **Less risk of dementia:** Scientists recently discovered a link between beta-amyloid accumulation in the brain and the development of dementia and Alzheimer's disease. As I discussed in chapter 4, beta-amyloid gets cleaned out of your brain in the deeper, slow-wave stages of sleep. When you miss out on deep sleep and log less than six hours a night, your brain doesn't get the nightly power wash it requires to stay healthy and function at its best—and as a result, your risk for developing dementia goes up by nearly 30 percent.[36] As the famous Bryan Adams said, "Let's Make a Night to Remember"—which in this context has a little more meaning than he planned for!

50. **Increased longevity:** If you sleep eight hours a night, does that guarantee you will live to be 100? No. Does wearing a seat belt ensure you won't be killed in a car accident? Also no. But both actions significantly increase your chances of a better outcome. The stats on this paint a bleak picture: When healthy adults get five hours or less a night, they have a threefold higher chance of dying within six years from that point.[37] Disorders like sleep apnea (breathing pauses at night) hack off about 7 to 10 years from your life. In addition to removing years from your life, they also remove the life from your years. Less sleep ups your chances for a faster death. So if you want to live your best, healthiest, longest, and happiest life possible, my advice is to protect your sleep tonight and every night thereafter.

Sleep Is First Class

You can see why sleep is one of the three pillars of good health: exercise, nutrition, and sleep. But I don't see them as equivalencies. I see sleep as different from the other two in a very important way: You don't have that little element of unhappiness that you sometimes get from disciplined nutrition (like giving up your favorite food if you're dieting) or exercise (pulling a hamstring in Pilates class). Sleep is unique in that you're not spending extra money on organic food if you're sleeping, you're not forcing yourself to crunch 50 sit-ups if you're sleeping, and you're not arguing with your spouse if you're sleeping. Sleep is one-third of your life, and it should be one of the best parts. To me, it's near perfect and as close to nirvana as you can get.

Using a plane analogy again, I like to think of sleep as first class. Nutrition is business class, and exercise is premium economy. Let's say that in your current life, you could do better. You know you need to make some changes to improve your health and well-being. You're sitting next to the restroom in economy class, in the seat that doesn't recline. There's a toddler kicking your seat from behind. You've been sitting on the tarmac for two hours already, and there's a long (cramped) journey ahead.

What if you could change seats right now, at this very moment? Your free upgrade to first class is just behind the curtain. There's a big, comfy seat set aside just for you.

What are you waiting for?

The Insomnia Connection

It's much harder to live a happy life when you're stressed out and sleep starved. It just is. I know this from talking to thousands of patients over the years . . . and I also know this from my own personal experience.

I'm a sleep physician, but that doesn't make me immune to the stressors of life shattering my own sleep at times. Before I got my green card, I endured almost two decades of uncertainty, mountains of paper work, and yes, many sleepless nights. And in the winter of 2020–21, my father in India came down with COVID. For six weeks, I worked long hours at the sleep clinic and lab, helped COVID patients at the local hospital, and somehow found time for my wife and daughter—all the while also taking phone calls at 2 a.m. from my father's doctor in India. (India is 10 and a half hours ahead of Indiana time.)

I felt horrible. I often lay awake at night with worry. And guess what happened? Cortisol, the stress hormone in my body, heightened. My sleep turned fragmented and poor. I stopped exercising, I was eating badly, I gained weight, I found myself not as productive as I wanted to be. I was short tempered at times, my mood darkened, and I completely neglected the activities I usually enjoy, like playing and making music. I can look back at this bleak time in my life and see what I was going through. It was short lived, thankfully. My dad healed from COVID, and the late-night phone calls ceased. My sleep pieced itself back together, and I found my happy once again.

Stress is a common cause of insomnia. And insomnia is a common risk factor for depression. My personal example shows how I swayed out of my sleep lane for a short time but corrected it soon enough. Most of us experience short-term insomnia like this, but it doesn't turn into a disorder.

But for others, it's different. Sometimes the stressors—financial, personal, emotional, what have you—persist, and if your brain is hardwired to go in that direction, that "little-i" insomnia (the symptom) can turn into "big-I" Insomnia (the disorder) as mentioned by Arizona sleep researcher and clinician Dr. Michael Grandner.

Three months is the boundary line. People who develop clinical insomnia often follow what we sleep physicians call the three P behavior model, a.k.a. the Spielman model: predisposition (a genetic factor, such as a family member with insomnia and the individual themselves being a light sleeper who is easily awakened), precipitating factor (a stressful life event like a birth, death, or job relocation), and perpetuation (the continuation of poor sleep habits, like lying in bed for hours trying to sleep when you're awake but can't fall asleep, long after the stressful precipitating factor has passed). These people are tired and wired, and their latent insomnia has risen up from below sea level to rear its ugly head.

I like to think of insomnia in terms of the Scoville Scale, which measures the heat of a pepper. Like a pepper, insomnia starts out mild and gets more intense. When we are born, we all start out as green peppers—these are lowest on the scale, at 0. But as you experience triggers in your life, your insomnia can get hotter and more severe. It might turn into a jalapeño (2,500–8,000), or it might become a superspicy habanero (100,000–350,000).

Treating insomnia is something of an art. You have to dis-cover the person's perpetuating factors and then untangle them. Are they extrinsic? Intrinsic? I need my patients to visu-alize this with me, and so I always draw it out for them on the paper covering the exam table. I scribble out their three Ps with my Sharpie, and they learn to see their insomnia in a new way.

My patient Audrey was a habanero. Well, technically she was a classical violinist diagnosed with classical insomnia. She was 29 but had experienced insomnia's onset at age 20, fol-lowing the death of her grandfather (the precipitating event) while she was in college. She complained of daytime fogginess, a low mood, and difficulty concentrating, and she struggled to fall or stay asleep. (Meanwhile, her husband complained about her grumpiness.) Her sleep schedule looked typical of an insomniac: in bed at 11 p.m. and up at 9 a.m., except for the occa-sional evening concert. Ten hours of "sleep"! Except she took an hour to fall asleep and woke up two to three times a night, and it often took her 30 minutes to several hours to fall back asleep. She slept very little, and sometimes she didn't sleep at all.

I told her about the three Ps, and she started cognitive behavioral therapy right away. Among other suggestions, I told her to restrict her sleep hours in bed to just six per day (to start). That way, she could experience a higher success rate in her sleep/wake ratio. I also recommended no caffeine after noon, no naps during the day, and a low dose of melatonin. The goal was to rev up her sleep drive.

Building up sleep drive is kind of like increasing water pressure behind a dam. When you first build the dam, the water is ankle height and not flowing well. The first five to six weeks of building up sleep drive—building the dam—are hard. But as the dam fills up and the water level rises, the pressure builds. Soon it will flow, and when the time is right, you can open the floodgates to sleep!

This analogy came to me after visiting the Bargi Dam on the Narmada River in India. I found myself watching the water and thinking about sleep in preparation for this chapter. Even when I'm on vacation, my sleep brain never sleeps!

Audrey followed my recommendations, and her sleep improved. By her first follow-up, she was sleeping a solid five and a half hours a night. By her second follow-up appointment, she reported she was able to fall asleep easily, and her sleep had extended to seven or so hours a night. She was a gold medal case for me. She hasn't needed to see me since then, and that was four years ago.

The harmful effects of poor sleep don't catch up with you right away. It's like a snowball rolling downhill. It starts out small but grows bigger and rolls faster. Except there's not just a snowball—there's an angry yeti chasing you too! We often can't "see" the damage sleep deprivation does to our bodies, so if it's easier, just imagine a yeti on a giant snowball gnashing his teeth and chasing you down a bumpy mountain of sleep. But don't surrender and lose all hope: The Sleep Vigilante is here to help you find your way to safety.

Sleep is essential for all of us, including babies, kids, and teens. In the next chapter, I dive into kids' sleep and why it's so important not only for their growing brains and bodies but also for the health, happiness, and well-being of the entire household. (I'd advise against sharing the yeti example with them: Even Bumble can be traumatizing to a five-year-old—just ask my coauthor.)

Chapter 6

The ABCs of Zzzs: Children's Health and Sleep

Sleep Vigilanteism: One child suffering
is the whole family suffering.

U p to this point, I've shared a lot of what I know about sleep, my experiences in the clinic, and even what the research says. I'm trained to help people sleep better—it's my life's passion, and I live and breathe sleep every single day . . . and night (no pun intended). So what happens when this same sleep physician (yours truly)—who has helped thousands of patients of all ages—brings his very own newborn baby home from the hospital? He gets her to sleep like an angel on a puffy cloud from day one, right?

Not even close, and you are absolutely correct if you guessed that all my training flew out the window the moment I laid our precious Baby Z* down in her bassinet in our room.

---

* Not her real name.

And when she started screaming, I became like every other frazzled new father before me: I had no idea what to do!

The pressure was on. The two things we worry about with babies are feeding and sleep. And as a trained sleep doc, I'm supposed to have 50 percent of that under control. Feeding was Mom's department; diaper duty and snooze duty were mine. I can tell you that being a sleep expert, everyone around me was semienvious that I had been trained in this. But surprise! Knee-deep in diapers and holding a squirming red-faced baby who could hit octaves I didn't even know existed, I faced an uncomfortable truth: I had no clue. I had lots and lots of training in the world of sleep but not so much in fatherhood. It's *so different* when it's your own baby. And so I started my on-the-job training in how to be a father and how to be my child's personal sleep doctor at the same time.

Back to Basics

I talk about this in chapter 1, but just to review, there are two processes we come preprogrammed with that we have little to no influence over, and those are the abilities to eat and to sleep. On the surface, they seem like activities we can control, but they are not. In fact, anytime we try to influence either one, it's mostly detrimental to the human species—like devouring doughnuts for breakfast every day for a month or taking sleep for granted on a regular basis, which so many of us do (the sleep part; hopefully not the doughnut part).

The cool thing about babies is they already know both of these processes. They're pros at eating and sleeping—you didn't teach them how; they just knew.

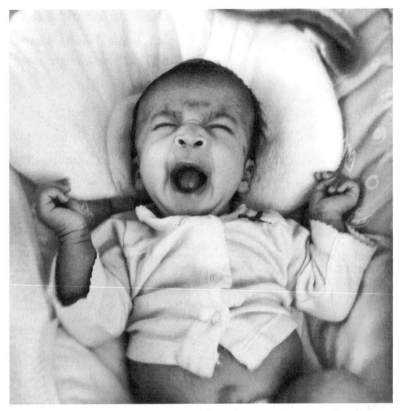

FIGURE 6.1. **Yawning or crying?** Thankfully, Baby Z was yawning in this precious moment, and all three of us (Mommy, baby, and me) took a nap right after. But lack of sleep can easily transform a peaceful image like this into a crying one, albeit one with a lot more decibels (crying for all: Mommy, baby, and me)!

Look at the picture of Baby Z (Fig. 6.1). I love this photo because you can't tell if she is yawning (because she is sleepy) or crying (because she is hungry). This picture encapsulates these two essential processes genetically programmed within all of us from the beginning. A baby's sleep-wake rhythm is so ingrained, in fact, that it develops inside the womb.

Once outside, these little bundles of joy now sleep (and fuss) in their parents' bedroom. With Baby Z curled up next to us in her bassinet, I began to think back to the basics of my sleep training and work toward establishing a healthy sleep pattern for my infant daughter. It wasn't easy, but as it turns out, she was a pretty decent sleeper (outside of her "off" days, which all babies have).

I'm going to share all my best tips (dare I call them "rules"?) in this chapter, but I'll also follow those up with a section on sleep disorders in children so you can know what healthy sleep looks like, recognize if one of the common sleep disorders may be affecting your child, and understand when it's time to seek help.

Before we get started, I want to share with you something foundational when it comes to children and sleep: the ideal number of hours needed to set them up for optimal health and success at every stage. (In case you are reading this book out of order, we talked in depth about sleep and its connection to success—including academic and athletic success—in chapter 3.) Believe me, you do not want your kid skimping on sleep!

The sleep needs of children evolve as they age, and sometimes it's hard to know if they're getting enough. To help you out, I've included a handy chart based on the latest sleep research, which was created by the sleep experts at the Sleep Foundation. You'll probably want to refer to this chart time and again as your child matures and grows toward adulthood. Let it be your guide. Knowing how much sleep your child actually needs (and doing all you can to keep them on track) is your first step in establishing a healthy sleep rhythm that is sure to be the envy of your entire neighborhood.

KIDS AND SLEEP: HOW MUCH DO THEY NEED?

AGE RANGE	RECOMMENDED HOURS OF SLEEP
Newborn (0–3 months)	14–17
Infant (4–11 months)	12–15
Toddler (1–2 years)	11–14
Preschool (3–5 years)	10–13
School age (6–13 years)	9–11
Teen (14–17 years)	8–10

Source: Eric Suni, "How Much Sleep Do We Really Need?," SleepFoundation.org, updated April 13, 2022, https://www.sleepfoundation.org/how-sleep-works/how-much-sleep-do-we-really-need.

Simple Sleep Plan for Kids

Every kid is unique, and the following sleep plan may need modification based on your lifestyle and your particular child. But consider it a good starting point for creating a plan that works for you and your family. Also keep reading for further ideas depending on your child's specific age.

If none of these suggestions seem to help your child sleep better—if you are following all the steps and still struggling—please seek the advice of an expert. Help *is* available. The sleep disorders section of this chapter (Sleep Disorders: Curiouser and Curiouser) will also help you make that determination.

Your child's brain and body are growing and repairing; they need their sleep to thrive. A ton of growth hormone is released when they are sleeping, so it's critical at all ages—infant, toddler, teen—that they log their required hours of sleep. Not to mention that no parent needs to be told what a poorly slept child looks like! Across all cultures, everyone knows. We've seen exhausted children on airplanes, on buses, and in grocery stores and heard them wailing from the apartment across the hall.

My simple sleep plan for kids is pretty straightforward. Just follow the six Ss:

1. *Same* bedtime and wake-up time each day (even on weekends)
2. *Screens* off two hours before bedtime
3. *Sweet spot* of 30 minutes for brushing teeth, PJs, snuggles, and story time
4. *Soothing* bedroom that is quiet, calm, dark, and a cool temperature of around 67°F or so
5. *Step out* of the room while they are still awake (and hopefully relaxed and drowsy) and before they fall asleep
6. *Structure* (Be as consistent as possible in your routine.)*

Is that an asterisk after #6? Yes! But why? Because although structure is so important—it's the Pavlovian classical conditioning that leads kids to good sleep routines; it's the set of events that compels a specific biological response (in this case, sleep)—you must also be flexible. (Not to mention that "six Ss and an F" doesn't quite have the same ring to it, does it?)

I got this idea of flexibility from one of my mentors, Dr. Steven Sheldon, a pediatric sleep medicine specialist in Chicago and a pioneer in the field. He would say, "Be consistent, persistent, and flexible." This applies beautifully to sleep in toddlers and school-age kids. You have to be consistent with the bedtime routine but also persistent. Children will push: one more song, one more book, one more kiss, one more sip of water, one more rhyme, one more hug. But you've got to set limits. No means no. Of course, don't let them cry it out. I'm not a big believer in that philosophy, especially in the beginning (as I will explain later in this chapter).

Flexibility means that when they are sick or when it's a weekend, you can delay their bedtime a little bit and watch a movie together, for example. As Dr. Sheldon says, "Flexible things bend; rigid things break."

A rigid sleep schedule can break everyone: the child breaks, you break, it's bad for the entire household. You don't want bedtime to become a wall you have to climb every night.

On the other hand, when childhood sleep schedules are flexible, they bend and remain unbroken. They help support a harmonious evening routine. And this routine is key. When you repeat it over and over, you form a circuit in the brain.

Special Considerations by Age

Now that you know my recommended sleep plan for kids, I want to dig a little deeper and mention a few additional suggestions, based on age, that I hope will help you even further. This section isn't all encompassing (I could probably write an entire book about children's sleep!), but it does highlight some common struggles parents tend to face.

Babies (0–11 months). Let's go back to my sweet Baby Z for a minute. I already knew that she needed 14 to 17 hours of sleep per day for optimal health. (I may have been exhausted, but my doctor brain still worked.) But how could we ensure that she got her best sleep? And for the sake of all bleary-eyed parents of newborns, how can you help your baby finally reach that golden milestone of sleeping through the night (hopefully sooner rather than later)?

For us, the answer to both of those questions was (at least in part) this: Baby Z would have her own bed from day one. She started out in a bassinet by our bed, but in just three weeks, she graduated to a crib in our bedroom. (That's what happens when you have a tall child whose long legs dangle precariously over the sides of the bassinet.) Then at age six weeks, we moved her into a crib in her own bedroom—equipped with a video baby monitor, a sound machine, and one of those timed light projectors that illuminate stars and baby sheep on the ceiling, of course.

Modern parents we were. Our decision to put Baby Z in her own bed to sleep clashed with the Indian culture my wife and I were both raised with as kids. In India, co-sleeping is the norm. Kids sleep with their parents until around age four, five, or six. The practice is common and acceptable; it is viewed as just a normal part of growing up.

But here we were, first-generation Indians in America, not doing that. And I will tell you, it was difficult for our parents to watch us breaking away from a tradition they hold dear. They questioned Baby Z's upbringing—"How can you do this? You should know better!" In their minds, putting Baby Z in her crib far away from us meant parental bonding was lost, irreparably. But as a sleep doctor, I knew there wasn't any science to support that. The research simply does not show that a child turns out worse or better due to co-sleeping. It's really about whatever works best for your situation. For us, we hoped that following this rule of training her to sleep alone in her own bed would benefit all of us (and our sleep). And I believe that it did. Baby Z met that milestone of sleeping through the night at just eight weeks, the earliest physiological age infants can do so, when their stomachs are finally big enough to stay full for a longer stretch of time.

Even though it can be hard at times to hold this boundary, the setup works especially well for working parents who need to protect their rest so they can stay alert on the job. You wouldn't want a pilot, surgeon, or air traffic controller with a baby or toddler at home to come to work sleep deprived!

Next, going back to step 5 in my "Simple Sleep Plan for Kids," you are going to try to step out of their room *before* they fall asleep. Put them down when they're drowsy, and let them see you walk away. Do not let them fall asleep while you're rocking or holding them; they need to feel comfortable with you leaving the room. This is so incredibly important! Because if you do not do this, *you* will also become an integral part of their routine, kind of like a pillow.

What do you do if your pillow falls out of position or off the bed in the middle of the night? You get up and reposition the pillow and fall right back to sleep, don't you? Leaving the child after they fall asleep is easier, but it makes you their "pillow." Then when they wake up in the middle of the night, they are unable to return to sleep easily because their favorite "pillow" (you) is missing. And so the child comes to associate you with the nightly bedtime setup, will not be able to fall asleep without you, and will barge into your bedroom at all hours once they're able to walk. Or they'll continually try to interrupt the rare Saturday-night movie you're trying to watch. Which leads us to . . .

Toddlers and preschoolers (1–5 years). Bedtime gets a bit hairy at this age because that little baby you could just swaddle and set down once upon a time has now become a short, mobile terror on two legs who would like nothing more than to turn the house upside down. That includes their sleep routine as well—they will do their very best to set fire to your nightly scheme and dance around the ashes in their diaper. Figuratively speaking, of course.

But don't let them. A common problem I hear from parents is that their children just keep leaving the bed after they've switched off the light and given the last goodnight kiss. They insist they're not tired! (And by the crazed look in their eyes, you just might believe them.) They just keep bolting out, little munchkin marathon runners with an insatiable need for your attention.

The first thing to do is play detective. Go back and reverse engineer the situation. Ask yourself the following questions:

- Why is your kid getting up in the middle of the night? Is something wrong with the routine?
- Are they sleeping too much during the day?
- Are you walking away when they are already asleep?
- Are they exposed to bright lights in the evening?
- Do they have a sleep disorder?
- Is there a recurring nightmare they are experiencing?
- Is the room too hot, too warm, or too cold at night?
- Are you continuing to feed the habit of them coming to your bed, crawling in, and sleeping in your bed with you? (If so, that becomes part of their sleep structure.)

If the structure is OK and consistent, yet they're still escaping out of their bed at night (ruining everyone's sleep from 2 a.m. to 6 a.m.), here's a trick I like to recommend, which I learned from Dr. Shalini Paruthi, a renowned pediatric sleep expert and codirector of the Sleep Medicine and Research Center at St. Luke's Hospital in St. Louis, Missouri, that she learned from her mentor, Dr. Timothy Hoban.

Tell little Liam that he gets two blue cards (or two items of your choice) at bedtime, but each time he runs out of the room, he loses a card. If he can keep both cards until morning, he gets a nice prize after he wakes up—it can be a Hot Wheels car, for example, or something else special he finds motivating. If he only has one card left at wake-up time, he can get a smaller prize—just make sure he sees what he *didn't* get. You can make the prize ceremony a big deal if you want—and make sure his siblings are watching too! The idea is to reinforce his choice to stay in his room. (Tell him that unless there is an emergency, there is no reason for him to come get you.) Once he learns how to succeed for one whole night, you can move the goalposts a little bit. Now it's *two* nights keeping the blue cards to get a prize and so on. After four weeks, the brain is wired, and you're done!

But what if Liam becomes inconsolable every time you put him back to bed? As I mentioned earlier, I don't believe in the "cry it out" method. But giving in, like so many parents do, isn't a solution either.

The secret here goes back to Dr. Sheldon's idea: Be flexible (mentioned earlier in this chapter). If you are too rigid, and if there is too much crying, they break . . . or you break. They aren't going to be in a positive mind space to learn to put themselves to sleep. Instead, what you can do is soothe them. Calm them down and reassure them. You can walk away, but it's OK to come back a few times if needed. You can even try a sleeping bag on the floor that gradually gets closer and closer to the door. You are being flexible, yes, but you are also continuing to extinguish the problem. Parents and kids really have to connect before an intervention takes place. Maybe try taking a long weekend, or a few days off work, to commit to this strategy so it's (quasi) painless.

School-age kids (6–13 years). With school-age kids, like Baby Z—who is now in elementary school (!!)—the same rules apply. The real problem I see at this age is reducing screen time and sticking to that ritual of no screens two hours before bed. The struggle is so hard for kids (and parents) that I've dubbed it World War Zzz!

Once screens are out of the picture, it also helps to limit sugar and choose natural snacks instead—foods with naturally occurring melatonin are a great choice if dinner was early and they want a little snack. (See "Sleep-Supporting Snacks" later in this chapter.) Also, keep the light exposure low as bedtime nears.

I also recommend you get *everyone* in sleep mode at the same time. At this age, kids don't want to miss out on any fun that Mom and Dad or big brother might be having once they're in bed. Rather, they want to be the center of attention and your evening. So make bedtime a shared experience. Have *everyone* in the household don their jammies, brush their teeth, and at least get ready for bed at the same time—your child will appreciate seeing that you are probably going to bed soon too. Make it a family ritual, and add in some bells and whistles, too, so that bedtime is super cozy—crack open *Harry Potter*, plug in the timed night-light, set the timer on the white noise machine, and so on.

Sleep-Supporting Snacks

The following foods are not just healthy—they also offer naturally occurring melatonin to support your child's sleep:

- cherries
- cucumber
- grapes
- kiwi
- oats
- peppers
- pistachios
- strawberries
- tomatoes

Source: X. Meng et al., "Dietary Sources and Bioactivities of Melatonin," *Nutrients* 9, no. 4 (2017): 367.

Teens (14–17 years). Teens are a different beast altogether. This is the age when they start to experience lots of changes—in their moods, hormones, bodies, social circles, impulses, and yes, even their sleep. In fact, this is the time of their life when we start to see what we call delayed sleep: Teens just naturally want to go to bed later at night and wake up later too. This tendency usually normalizes in their 20s (phew!), but it explains why they're so often zonked out until noon on a Saturday.

Why does this happen? We don't know for sure, but Dr. Mary Carskadon, adjunct professor of cognitive, linguistic, and psychological sciences and professor of psychiatry and human behavior at Brown University in Providence, Rhode Island, described the following theory in a National Academy of Sciences presentation: She hypothesized that their body clocks are naturally delayed because we, as a species, have always had to protect ourselves from predators. And so the younger and healthier among us could do the graveyard shift, scare away hungry saber-toothed cats, and protect the elderly, who naturally fall asleep earlier. By the time the young teenagers fell asleep, it would be time for the elderly to get up and take over their shift (say 4 or 5 a.m.). Also by this time, the predators would be asleep, and the elderly would have an easier time guarding. It's called herd theory, and teen sleep patterns made a lot more sense when we lived in caves. But now, when swim practice starts at 6 a.m. and the school bell rings at 8, it feels like a square peg in a round hole.

The problem isn't just that it's hard to drag our teenage kids out of bed in the morning. It's more serious than that: When teens don't get enough sleep, they're not just cranky—their academics suffer and they start to show signs of anxiety, depression, and even attention deficit hyperactivity disorder (ADHD). Now factor in high exposures to blue wavelength light, which is emitted from screens, phones, and video games. Blue light suppresses melatonin, activates the brain, and makes falling asleep that much more difficult.

Some forward-thinking high schools (increasing in number both nationally and internationally), following the science and hoping for a better-rested student body on the whole, have moved morning start times later to account for this. Whether or not this is the case for your district, you can support your child by scheduling activities later in the morning on weekends and not pressuring them to carry too heavy a schedule that steals the sleep they so desperately need.

That's assuming, of course, that your child's sleep patterns fall into the normal range. If you suspect something deeper is happening—perhaps even a sleep disorder—continue reading the next section, which focuses on the most common sleep disorders affecting kids and teens and highlights important warning signs.

Sleep Disorders: Curiouser and Curiouser

When Ava, a 14-year-old athlete, and her dad came to my office for help, it was clear right away that something was very wrong. I soon learned that she tossed and turned and stared at the clock every night until 2 a.m., and she also had difficulty waking up in the morning. On weekends, she had no problem sleeping from 3 a.m. until noon uninterrupted. But her grades sank lower than normal. She wasn't performing well in her sport. And she appeared to be borderline depressed.

They'd tried everything, but nothing worked. Her family and doctor wondered, Did she have ADHD? Was it just regular teenage hormones and angst? Her pediatrician tried treating her for big-I Insomnia (the disorder), so she'd been consuming a concoction of over-the-counter meds, sleep aids, and even a medication not officially approved for use in children. And yet no improvement.

Once I met with her, it occurred to me that this might not be Insomnia after all. There is a common sleep disorder in kids that *looks* like Insomnia, but it's not. (You may remember from chapter 5 that when insomnia is just a symptom, it can be called "small-i" insomnia. Insomnia the disorder, by contrast, can be thought of as "big-I" Insomnia. "Small-i" insomnia, if left untreated and repeated for long enough, can turn into actual Insomnia.)

The disorder I was able to diagnose Ava with, following our standard sleep medicine clinic evaluation, is called **delayed sleep-wake phase disorder**, and it's one of the most common sleep disorders we see in teens. In delayed sleep-wake phase disorder, the time a child is able to naturally fall asleep at night is delayed by hours beyond the normal time they should be falling asleep. But once they fall asleep, they're able to stay asleep just fine. I told Ava that her brain and body clocks were on California time, yet she was living in Indiana (Eastern Time). I joked that if she just moved to Los Angeles, her sleep would be perfect. Delayed sleep-wake phase disorder happens to be a very common sleep arrhythmia that often goes unnoticed and is mislabeled with other diagnoses.

I put together a comprehensive sleep plan for her to follow over summer break. (It can take up to four weeks to move your internal clock and synchronize it with the external clock.) She used bright-light therapy in the mornings and melatonin at night to slowly (15 minutes every three days or so) move her sleep-wake rhythm to Indiana time. These are tiny increments of time I'm talking about. It's like the slow *click-click-click* that happens when you dial a safe or turn a ship's direction. At some point, it will click into the right spot, and the door will open (or the direction will be corrected). The treasure inside is refreshing, incredible sleep—the kind we all dream of!

A few months later, Ava and her father followed up with me. Overjoyed, they shared the wonderful news: She was sleeping well, was no longer depressed, her grades had climbed back up, she'd gotten off all the meds, and she was back in sports, feeling strong. These kinds of magical moments really are the best parts of my job.

Another interesting case that came to me was that of Nicole, a bright 17-year-old student just about ready to graduate and go to college. When I first met her, she complained of being very sleepy, was not doing well in school, and said she was sleeping in the night *and* had the irresistible urge to sleep during the day. She experienced hallucinations at the edge of wake and sleep too: Sometimes she saw spiders crawling down her arm or shadows of people walking past her. She and her primary care doctor both wondered what was going on. He thought at first that she might have a mood disorder, but then he had the good idea to send her to a sleep doc: me.

I conducted a sleep test and voilà! Without a doubt, Nicole had narcolepsy! (The most positive, unambiguous sleep study result of narcolepsy you could ever imagine.) It feels so good to know what the problem is because then we can treat it. With this disorder, the edges of sleep and wake get a little fuzzy. Despite getting an adequate quantity of sleep at night, the sufferer zones out into little microsleeps, including dream/REM sleep, usually without their awareness (which explains the hallucinations). But the lack of quality sleep builds up over time, and they end up feeling terrible.

Imagine that inside your body is a sleep switch. When you flip it up, it stays that way for 18 hours (the time you are awake), and then it falls slowly down (for sleep) due to gravity. And then after getting your 8 hours of sleep, the switch flips back up again and is ready for the day. That is how it is for those of us with normal, healthy sleep. But with narcoleptics, that switch is floppy. Even when the switch is up, it keeps wanting to fall back down into sleep mode all day long.

Although narcolepsy is treatable, there is no cure for the disorder—yet. But thankfully, with our tailored treatment plan and the right balance of medications, Nicole is back at school, performing well academically, and grateful to be back to her normal self.

It's kind of a mystery, but with Nicole's case (and perhaps many others), her narcolepsy likely was present for nearly a decade. But it wasn't until her later teenage years that it worsened to the point where she actually noticed it and experienced its negative impacts.

Most Common Sleep Disorders in Kids and Teens

As you can see, I run across all kinds of sleep disorders in my clinic. And so I thought it would be helpful to round up the top disorders that seem to affect kids the most, in case it can be of help to you, your family, or someone close to you. Take a look, and if any of the following descriptions feel a little bit familiar, I encourage you to seek the advice of a sleep specialist.

Sleep Disorder: Behavioral Insomnia of Childhood: "Big-I" Insomnia (as mentioned earlier in this chapter)
Typical age of onset: Toddlers and up
Signs to look for:
- difficulty falling and staying asleep
- occurs more than three days a week for three months

Sleep Disorder: Delayed Sleep-Wake Phase Disorder: As discussed in the previous section, the child, typically in the adolescent age group, is not able to fall asleep at a regular hour, and sleep onset is delayed by several hours. Many times, the child is not able to fall asleep until past midnight. But once they fall asleep, they are able to stay asleep just fine.

Typical age of onset: Adolescence

Signs to look for:

- difficulty falling asleep or waking up at socially acceptable or required times
- difficulty staying awake in the daytime
- irritability
- "small-i" insomnia

Sleep Disorder: Hypersomnia or Narcolepsy: Excessive sleepiness during the day

Typical age of onset: Preteens (could be earlier in a few) and onward

Signs to look for:

- difficulty staying awake during the day despite adequate nighttime sleep quantity
- hallucinations, frequently visual at the time of waking or falling asleep
- zoning out
- sleep paralysis: inability to move upon waking
- irresistible episodes of sleepiness
- muscle weakness (such as knees buckling) with a strong emotion such as laughter

Sleep Disorder: Parasomnia: Night terrors, sleep talking, sleepwalking, nightmares

Typical age of onset: Young children. These tend to reduce in frequency as the young brain matures and its neural wiring managing sleep and wake also matures and these two states interfere less with each other.

Signs to look for:

- significant daytime impact: sleepiness in the daytime, lack of focus, napping, feeling tired (if this is the case, it's a great idea to reach out to their doc and discuss options)

Sleep Disorder: Restless Sleep Disorder (RSD): RSD is a new disorder just identified in 2020.[1] The child will thrash around, kick, and fall out of bed at night during sleep.

Typical age of onset: Age six and older

Signs to look for:

- five or more large body movements per hour
- daytime crankiness
- behavior problems

Sleep Disorder: Sleep Apnea and Snoring: For brief moments, the child will stop breathing during sleep.

Typical age of onset: Toddlers and up

Signs to look for:

- snoring noises during sleep, with or without intermittent breathing pauses followed by recovery gasps (in young children, snoring can be difficult to hear)
- restless sleep
- irritability during the day
- excessive daytime sleepiness
- bed-wetting (at times)

The abovementioned sleep disorders in kids are common and even more commonly left untreated. Unfortunately, these are critical years for a child's development, and untreated sleep disorders likely have a significant impact much beyond what we can measure. We must wake up *right now* to the importance of sleep.

Now that we've had our primer on kids and sleep, let's move on to the next age group we need to talk about: aging adults in their golden years, 65-plus. (Even if you think this doesn't apply to you right now, it may apply to someone you love.) But before you turn the page, there is one takeaway I want to leave you with: The better the child sleeps, the happier the family will be.

A Dangerous Diagnosis?

We have to be careful when diagnosing ADHD and anxiety in kids. In my practice, about one-third of the hyperactive kids I see actually just have a sleep disorder. The problem is, when doctors look for that quick fix and scribble out a prescription, yes, they're treating the symptoms and the child seems to calm down, but the underlying issue—lack of quality sleep—frequently remains unaddressed.

When doctors fail to solve the actual problem, kids suffer and spend their childhood on medications unnecessarily. But once you fix their sleep (assuming that is indeed the problem), they can feel bright and calm and be their best selves again. And you can eliminate the need for unnecessary meds!

Warning Signs Your Child Is Not Getting Enough Sleep

- tantrums
- hyperactivity
- overeating
- behavior problems
- learning problems
- falling asleep in class
- grades dropping

Is Your Child an Owl or a Lark?

You may have heard this analogy before: If your child is an owl, he likes to stay up later and sleep in. If she's a lark, she wants to go to bed early and rise early too. Pay attention to your kid's natural tendencies, and you can then identify the right individualized bedtime / wake time that works best for them.

Chapter 7

Aging, and Sleeping, Gracefully

Sleep Vigilanteism: Good quality sleep will add more years to your life—and more life to your years.

Marilyn was in her early 70s when her sleep began to deteriorate. She experienced a litany of upsetting symptoms: insomnia, daytime tiredness, frequent middle-of-the-night wake-ups, dry mouth, low mood, and the urge to use the bathroom four times a night. Her urologist couldn't find anything wrong, but he wondered if, as the mom of five kids, her numerous pregnancies had altered her anatomy enough to lead to incontinence. Interestingly, though, her frequent urination habit did not occur during the day—only at night. Something didn't add up.

Her doctor figured she might have insomnia, and so she went on sleeping pills. This is almost always the first thing sleep sufferers reach for, but it is usually not the best long-term solution. She hadn't yet uncovered the underlying reason for her problem, and the meds weren't helping either. Eventually, Marilyn showed up in my office seeking advice and solutions.

As she sat across from me and listed her symptoms, I soon learned that Marilyn had no trouble falling asleep—and yet a hallmark of garden variety insomnia is that you cannot fall asleep; your mind can't slow down enough for you to fall asleep. I asked her, "Do you snore?" She didn't think so (and her husband, who had died a few years ago, had never mentioned it). She also revealed she took three pills a day to help her sleep: a bladder pill, a sleeping pill, and an antidepressant. After completing a physical exam of her oral and airway anatomy and considering all parts of her health history, I put her through a sleep study. The result? Moderate sleep apnea.

Many people associate sleep apnea with obesity, but it doesn't exclusively occur in someone who is overweight. Also, sleep apnea can present differently in older adults. Marilyn is a case in point: She was larger built but in the normal weight range for height—not thin, but not overweight either. Also, she probably didn't snore very loudly. My guess is she likely always had a mild case of sleep apnea but didn't notice it until she went through menopause and put on a few extra pounds. Both of these factors made her sleep apnea worse.

She started a CPAP regimen and began to feel better. (For more on CPAP devices and how far they've come since their invention in the early 1980s, see chapter 9.) I like CPAP machines because they are an effective, nonpill, nonsurgical way of treating a sleep disorder. As for Marilyn? She soon felt like her cheerful and well-rested self again, she no longer needed naps in the day, and her nighttime bathroom breaks dwindled to just one. Even better, she was able to stop all three of those pills she'd been taking in a misguided attempt to improve her sleep. Here she was in her 70s, sleeping wonderfully yet again.

The Sleep and Aging Myth

There's this myth about sleep and aging that says you can't experience quality sleep once you've reached a certain age. I don't believe this to be true: I say you can age gracefully and learn to sleep gracefully too. Will there be challenges? Yes. But they can be overcome.

Sometimes I tell my patients to think of a BMW: This well-made car will run just fine at 200,000 miles with the right care. Of course, you have to service it on a regular basis and address any issues as they arise. You can't expect it to last if you neglect to take care of it diligently. However, with the right attention, the car drives great even after it zooms past the 100,000-mile mark (and even further down the road).

Your body works much the same way: It's beautifully made, but you must attend to the regular service of it through diet, exercise, and—most importantly—sleep if you want it to continue to take you where you need to go well into your 60s, 70s, and beyond. Poor sleep, like poor maintenance on a car, will ding little bits and pieces of every part of your body, head to toe. Sleep touches everything.

Navigating Change

According to the Administration for Community Living, about 21 percent of the U.S. population will be over age 65 by 2040.[1] That's a huge number of people I hope will pay more attention to their sleep as they age. If you're over age 65 right now, you may be feeling some of sleep's natural, expected changes.

Delta waves. In chapter 4, I talked about delta waves and their vital role in cleansing your brain during deep low-wave sleep. We've all experienced this: When you obtain the nourishing balance of REM and NREM complements, it's the best kind of sleep. You wake up feeling refreshed, and it's easier to get into these deeper sleep states when you're young.

Unfortunately, these powerful sleepy-time brain waves diminish as we age. We can measure them in older adults and see the data right there in black and white that as we get older, we just don't log as much deep sleep. Those big, comforting delta waves become fewer and fewer.

Why? We don't really know. More importantly, can we get them back? Again, we're not quite sure. Scientists are researching delta waves and studying if we can encourage them or give them a little boost to promote more refreshing sleep.

I find this idea of "sleep engineering" fascinating. What if we could promote delta sleep waves and keep them strong our whole life? There is a theoretical possibility that doing so could bring major advantages to memory, growth, repair, and so on. (You can read more about brain waves during sleep and their probable correlation to Alzheimer's and dementia in chapter 4.) We don't have all the answers (yet), but it's an exciting frontier of study with tantalizing possibilities.

Reduced melatonin production. In addition to these precious delta waves floating further and further out of our grasp, the pineal gland in your brain also begins to produce less melatonin, the sleep hormone. In simple terms, this natural change makes it harder to sleep as deeply as you did when you were younger.

Sleep fragmentation. This means you are more easily awakened by interruptions that 20 or 30 years ago you could just snooze through. Once you hit your 60s and beyond, you may start to notice you wake up more frequently in the night, and you struggle more than usual to fall back to sleep too. These nighttime interruptions lead to more daytime naps and can become a vicious cycle. We call this kind of broken sleep "fragmentation."

Even more painful jet lag. Remember in your 20s and 30s, when flying across time zones and readjusting your sleep was just a minor inconvenience that was easily corrected? Not so now. Older adults often have a much harder time resetting their sleep schedules following this kind of abrupt disruption. And so that Los Angeles–London trip you've waited all year for is going to wreak more havoc on your sleep schedule than anticipated. Missing sleep for a late Saturday-night social activity will be harder to adjust to as well.

Your two vital sleep systems change. As I mentioned in the previous chapter, when discussing herd theory and the thinking behind why teens desire to stay up past midnight, the opposite begins to happen to the elders of the household: They reach a certain age and find themselves nodding off several hours earlier than they did in their prime. And now they're waking up like roosters at 5 a.m. too!

As you age, the two intertwined systems that regulate your sleep just don't work as robustly as they once did: your master clock (a.k.a. circadian rhythm), which responds to light and dark cycles, and your homeostatic system, which regulates that delicate balance between sleep and wake. This can be upsetting to someone who is accustomed to being a night owl and now falls asleep in a chair every afternoon before dinner.

This isn't usually a problem unless the change is so extreme that it begins to interfere with your normal social activities. Are you unable to stay awake through dinner? Are you too tired to pick your grandkids up after softball practice? Do you wake up, wide-eyed, at 3 a.m.? You may have advanced sleep-wake phase disorder, and this disorder can be rectified with treatment that includes synchronizing your internal clock back with the sun a little bit better, using a light box, and other therapies under the guidance of a sleep physician.

Age-related ailments. As if that wasn't enough, many older adults also typically contend with health ailments, arthritis, pain, and discomfort, all of which affect sleep negatively. Some of the drugs they take, too, interfere with sleep—from antidepressants, blood pressure pills, and water pills to pain meds and muscle relaxers. Always talk to your doc about what you're taking and its potential side effects. (Not to mention that over-the-counter sleeping pills can inter-act with these meds too!) It's OK to ask if a medication will mess with your sleep and what you can do to counteract that.

You should also consult the AGS Beers Criteria from the American Geriatrics Society (easily found online), which lists common drugs—including antihistamines and sleeping pills—considered potentially unsafe for seniors. Aging bodies process medications differently compared to when they were young, so something you used to take in your 30s might not be safe for you now.

The Hidden Dangers of Sleeping Pills

Sleeping pills may be used in moderation for a short time and ideally under the guidance of a physician, but when used frequently or routinely or for longer periods, older adults are putting themselves at risk for the following:

- possible serious interactions with other medications
- increased risk of falls
- impaired balance
- memory loss
- daytime drowsiness
- reduced deep sleep states

When you take all of these uncomfortable life changes into consideration, it's no wonder that sleep in your later years gets such a bum rap. This does *not* mean you are destined to suffer terrible sleep for the remainder of your life. The road to sleep may be riddled with more potholes, sure, but if you drive with caution, you can avoid some of the biggest ones and be less affected by those you do encounter.

Improving Your Sleep . . . sans Pills

Despite all of the above interferences, older adults still need their requisite seven to eight hours of sleep per night for brain and body health and well-being. My strategies in chapter 10,

"The Easy Sleep Reset," compose a great daily plan for everyone, and I suggest you start there. But I'm also including some additional tips here to offset the natural changes (and alas, setbacks) you're bound to face as you age. (I hope you'll notice I'm offering tried-and-true behavioral solutions that *don't* require you to reach for that half-empty bottle of sleeping pills at your bedside.) This list isn't exhaustive, but it highlights some of the most common ones and how to adapt.

Excessive napping. I mentioned earlier how sleep fragmentation can lead to daytime napping, which causes more fragmented sleep, and so on. You can stop the vicious cycle by setting a 30-minute alarm on your phone if you feel the need to take a nap. You still get that little bit of rest your body craves, but you're not getting so much that your nighttime sleep becomes a struggle. As I mention throughout this book, napping can be healthy for you—but there is that risk of too much of a good thing.

Dietary sleep disruptors. Just like napping too much can ruin your sleep, so can wine, sugar, caffeine, tobacco, and eating dinner less than three hours before bedtime. They act like darts in the balloons of sleep. These kinds of indulgences don't noticeably bother your body and sleep as much when you're young, and adapting to change can sometimes be hard for older people.

Nighttime bathroom breaks. Staying hydrated is important, but don't drink lots of water before bed—keep your hydration up throughout the day instead. Also, avoid diuretics (such as medications for high blood pressure) at night if possible; they increase your need to urinate, so schedule them for in the morning or earlier in the day instead. If you're diabetic (or even if you're not), don't pry open that tub of Ben & Jerry's right before bed. Your pancreas and bladder (and sleep!) will thank you.

Men versus women. As men and women age, they each face unique challenges when it comes to sleep. Women face hormonal problems, hot flashes, and sleep fragmentation thanks to menopause; meanwhile, men have to deal with enlarged prostates, which cause frequent urination. Sometimes lifestyle changes, like restricting fluids in the evening (for men), wearing breathable pajamas (for women), and reducing stress and following a healthy sleep routine (for both), are all that are needed.

Both men and women also face an increased risk of sleep apnea in their later years—though it affects men more than women. This disorder isn't something you can self-diagnose; you'll need the input and guidance of a trained sleep physician. The increased risk may also be due to the fact that sleep apnea in women often presents differently than in men and can often go unnoticed for longer. (I speak more about sleep apnea later in this chapter and throughout the book.)

Less sunlight. I don't want to generalize here, but the aging adults I see in my clinic tend to be less active outdoors in sunlight in their later years. Their schedules, responsibilities, abilities, and interests just aren't what they used to be: They aren't chasing a giggling four-year-old across the playground; they're not shooting hoops with friends after school; because of hip pain, they're not power walking around the block anymore; they're depressed and unmotivated because their kids and grandkids haven't visited in eight months.

Whatever the reason may be, life slows down, and someday your routine changes to the point where you just aren't soaking up as much sunlight as you once did.

This may seem like a minor thing, but lack of sunlight impacts your ability to sleep big time. Getting out in the sun every single day (preferably in the morning, before lunch) is vital to the proper function of your circadian rhythm. Activity in sunlight boosts your mood too. Depending on your situation, you may need to think creatively here—but getting active outdoors is a huge determinant of how well you're going to sleep at night.

I advise all my older patients to prioritize healthy sun exposure as much as possible in their daily routines. Do whatever you can to keep your social calendar full. Tend to your garden. Eat lunch alfresco. Play some tennis. Make moving your body a priority, even if it's just for 20 minutes a day. Exercising plus feeling the sun on your skin will rev up your sleep *and* wake drives! Just try it—you will experience the benefits firsthand.

A word about exercise: This can feel like an overwhelming ask for older adults with certain health problems. But keep in mind, when I say "exercise," it doesn't have to mean running for 30 minutes down a California beach. It can come in different forms, and it's OK to tailor it to your abilities as needed. Maybe it means simple chair exercises. Maybe you stand for 30 minutes while watching TV instead of sitting. Perhaps you can park farther away from your destination so you can kick your heart rate up.

The Magnificent Seven-in-One Pill

IMAGINE A LIFE-CHANGING PILL OF
SEVEN MEDICATIONS ROLLED INTO ONE.

My favorite thing about exercise is that it's a powerful sleep promoter. But it's also beneficial for overall health. I like to think of daily exercise as a magic pill with seven magnificent medications rolled into one:

1. Antianxiety pill
2. Antihypertensive
3. Heart pill
4. Cholesterol pill
5. Diabetes pill
6. Antidepressant / mood booster
7. Sleeping pill (the most important part!)

Your body loves a schedule, and this is especially important if you are retired and the days and weeks just stretch out before you with nothing exciting circled on the calendar. Get up at 8 a.m., go for a walk, soak up some sun, grab coffee or lunch with a friend—and at night, go to bed at a set time. Take ownership of your days and stick to your routine. Your body thrives on this kind of repetition (and so does your sleep).

If lack of mobility is causing depression (or vice versa), you've got to break the cycle somehow so you can feel better.

Talk to your doctor. Lean on your social support if needed. You may need an exercise trainer or an antidepressant under the guidance of a physician. Moving your body more means sleeping better—which in turn gives you more energy during the day.

Could It Be a Sleep Disorder?

If nothing seems to work—you're getting sunlight, you're following my Four-Play Method for sleep in chapter 10, you're eliminating all the major sleep disruptors, and you're generally in good health—the obvious question becomes, Do you have a sleep disorder?

Insomnia is a common one in this age group, especially in menopausal women, as noted in the SWAN (Study of Women's Health across the Nation) study, among others.* Meet Tracy, a patient of mine in her late 50s who was experiencing overall terrible sleep. She had gained a little weight after menopause, and her sleep had become fragmented. Her doctor discussed taking hormones, but due to her history of breast lumps, they decided against it. She then went on a low dose of Prozac. Her mood improved, but her sleep got even worse! She found herself jolting awake with night sweats and uncomfortable restless limb movements.

Frustrated and overwhelmed by lack of sleep, she came to see me. A few things stood out right away as we talked: First, she obsessively checked the clock all night and got stressed as

---

* The SWAN study is cosponsored by the National Institute on Aging, the National Institute of Nursing Research, the National Institutes of Health, the Office of Research on Women's Health, and the National Center for Complementary and Alternative Medicine.

the minutes slowly ticked by. Second, she had fallen into this habit of unloading the dishwasher, eating snacks, and folding clothes in the middle of the night when her insomnia got bad. And third, she magically slept just fine in a hotel or at a friend's house.

Insomnia often has a strong psychological component, and so it was interesting to me that she slept great everywhere except her own bed. I determined she needed to engage in cognitive behavioral therapy to fix her nightly routine. She also needed to reestablish positive associations with bedtime and unlearn the aversion she had developed to her own bedroom. It was almost like as soon as bedtime fell, she found herself entering a boxing ring instead of a cozy, peaceful bed, and she anticipated losing the fight every night to her unstoppable opponent: insomnia.

I looked at all aspects and aimed to remove every maladaptation that had become so ingrained. I encouraged her to follow a new set of rules: for example, no checking the clocks or folding laundry when she couldn't sleep. After a discussion with her prescribing physician, I slowly weaned her off the Prozac.

It took about two months, but after that, she was doing a whole lot better. Her three to four awakenings per night decreased to just one, and she no longer needed my help. I like to think that a well-treated insomnia patient should never have to see me again. If I lose a patient, the patient wins because they've gained their sleep back!

Maybe you, too, have developed aversions to sleep. If your budget allows, you can even go a step further and redesign your bedroom so it feels like a fresh space. It's a helpful visual reminder that you're not in the boxing ring anymore. It's amazing what a coat of paint (in a calming color like a soft blue, beige, green, or pink), rearranged pictures or new art, and crisp, new bed linens can do to make you feel a renewed sense of harmony.

A Hard Habit to Break

One of the worst aspects of insomnia is that you can get into this habit of overthinking and worrying at night, jumping from thought to thought, spinning your wheels—and the problem just perpetuates itself. Insomnia carves an unpleasant but familiar groove into your mind, and eventually, every night becomes just as bad as (or worse than) the one before. Night after night, you lay awake thinking about how bad your day is going to be, and sleep just drifts further and further out of reach, and you slowly sink deeper into the quicksand of sleeplessness. Before you know it, two years have gone by, and you're relying on prescription sedatives just to get some shut-eye. The cycle repeats for months, years—sometimes even decades.

So many of my patients wash, rinse, and repeat insomnia night after night after night. They actually get *good* at sleeping poorly! That's because our bodies are quite effective at mastering any repetitive activity—you can get good at eating an unhealthy diet; you can get good at slumping at your desk.

Insomnia is like a bad knot on a big, fat rope. It's hard to undo the knot. Even if you succeed, the kink is still there. But if you give it a few weeks to a couple of months, the kink slowly goes away.

I help my patients undo that knot and train into a good habit. We find the right series of positive behaviors to repeat, and instead of insomnia, they slowly start to get wonderful sleep. You can start this training in your 50s and 60s—it's never too late to learn. It's like going to the gym: You don't build muscles in just one day. It takes day after day of repetitive exercises to start to see results. It's the same with sleep.

That said, I do encounter a situation unique to the population of adults 65-plus: Their insomnia habit can be so far gone, it's been cemented in for decades. The knot on their rope is tighter, it's harder to undo, and the kink stays around a lot longer once you work it out. There are no easy fixes here. These people have to work harder to realign their sleep. But even then, it can be done. It just takes a lot more patience, belief in the process, and commitment.

That's why I encourage people not to wait too long to see a trained physician if they're experiencing serious sleep issues. It's much easier to intervene in a bad habit before the cement cures. My hope is that this book spurs readers of all ages—whether in their 20s or 60s—to get help if needed and fix any issues early before poor sleep settles in.

I'm so glad Tracy walked into my office when she did, while still in her 50s. Her solutions were simple and took just eight weeks to yield results. Imagine if she had suffered from insomnia like that for 20 more years—how much harder it would have been for us to assemble a solution! She would have been miserable, aged poorly, and not lived her last few decades well.

Listen to Your Heart

As a sleep physician, I've almost begun to develop a sixth sense when it comes to diagnosing sleep disorders. And when I begin to suspect something's going on, oftentimes my patients push back a little. They say, "No, Doc, I'm fine. I don't think I have *that* problem." Sometimes it takes a whole lot of convincing from me to persuade my reluctant patients to take a simple sleep test.

This was the case with Cruz, an otherwise fit and healthy 75-year-old man who had started suffering from atrial fibrillation (or A-fib), a common heart rhythm problem in the 65-plus crowd. He initially controlled it pretty well with a common heart and blood pressure medication, but his doctor sent him to me because he had started waking up in the night with a racing, pounding heart plus intermittent palpitations during the day—all of which were tracked and recorded on the heart monitor his cardiologist had him wear. But perhaps even more upsetting, Cruz found himself breathless on the golf course and unable to play his favorite game. (Up until this point, he normally hit the green five days per week.) He also admitted to falling into long naps in the day and filling up on extra sugary drinks just to keep his tired eyes open.

His quality of life was spiraling down the drain—yet it was hard for this retired engineer to believe that he could possibly have a sleep problem when he was pretty sure it was just a heart problem.

Thankfully, he had come to the Sleep Vigilante, and I was confident I knew what was going on. After our initial consultation, I suggested we evaluate him in our sleep lab overnight, a request that (as mentioned earlier) didn't go over too well at first. He did comply (with reluctance, I might add), and indeed my suspicions were confirmed.

The man suffered from moderate sleep apnea.

He wasn't obese, he didn't have a thick neck, his wife wasn't elbowing him in the middle of the night for roaring snores—he didn't show any of those "classic signs" of sleep apnea you might see when trying to self-diagnose on Google. But I've seen patients like him before, and as I showed you earlier with Marilyn, the very first case study to open this chapter, sleep apnea presents differently in older adults. But this mystery can be solved when you know what to look for.

Our lab captured Cruz's heart abnormalities, which occurred alongside each sleep apnea event. With every episode, he lost airflow and his body panicked a little, which revved up his heart. He then stopped breathing for several seconds, and the body responded by releasing adrenaline. He'd then wake up with a racing heart, and the scenario played out again and again, night after night. This explains why he (and other sleep apnea sufferers like him) felt so terrible every day.

Even after all this, Cruz still didn't believe he had sleep apnea, and he balked at my treatment plan. "Just try a little CPAP," I told him (and many others before him too). "You don't have anything to lose!" No one ever wants to start using a CPAP device. Begrudgingly, he complied, and so I fitted him with his device.

I think you can probably guess how this story ends.

In just six weeks, he felt so much better. After a few tweaks and a few interface changes, he learned to tolerate the CPAP device just fine—in fact, he came to welcome it because he got his normal energy and life back! He is back to his golf game, he's no longer napping or chugging Sprites all day, and he's not scaring himself awake with heart palpitations in the night. The last time I met with him, he said he was talking with his cardiologist about lowering some of his heart medications. Which is really amazing if you think about it! Sleep is so powerful a medicine that it can *become* your medicine. And help heal, I daresay, anything.

I hate to imagine what might have been had he *not* fixed his sleep. He would have stopped a lot of physical activity and lost his independence. He would have needed more meds, maybe required surgical procedures (heart ablations), and perhaps experienced difficult side effects. He would have lost his beloved hobby forever and probably sunken into a depression. But thanks to better-quality sleep, he gained more life in his years. (If that sounds a bit familiar, think back to my Sleep Vigilanteism that opened this chapter.)

The Sleep Apnea Crisis

A lot of the examples in this book call attention to sleep apnea. It's by design: My feeling is that it can never be talked about enough. Sleep apnea is dangerous if left untreated and at the same time is extremely common—about one in five to six adults suffer from it—and yet, of those, only 10 to 20 percent get diagnosed, according to the American Academy of Sleep Medicine. The rest go undiagnosed or untreated and suffer serious health consequences—slowly but surely!

Using the BMW example from earlier, sleep apnea is kind of like when one of your wheels is out of alignment, and it keeps wobbling your car as you drive. No matter how many times you hammer it back into place, it keeps wobbling until you fix the underlying problem—in this case, sleep apnea is like a broken or missing bolt. If you continue to drive the car in this condition of disrepair, you might get by in the short term. But doing so is detrimental to the long-term viability of your car—or in this case, your body.

When sleep apnea is an underlying disorder related to another devastating health problem, like my patient Cruz and his heart issues, treating it is especially important. The Heart Rhythm Society reports that about 50 percent of A-fib patients also have sleep apnea. But if ignored, sleep apnea increases the failure of A-fib treatments by two to three times![2] When interventions for A-fib fail, we're talking heart failure and stroke. On the plus side, awareness seems to be rising: Every single week, I see five patients sent over from the heart rhythm clinic. Now multiply that by those seen by my partners and other sleep physicians nationwide too. Hopefully, all people (not just older adults) are ready to wake up to this risk.

Investing in your sleep will never hurt anything; in fact, it will always net a positive impact on your life. And no matter your age, it's never too late to make positive changes. I've never heard a patient tell me they feel miserable after sleeping better!

Just as I listen to my patients with my heart, I ask that you listen to your heart too. It may be telling you it's time to talk to your primary care doc at your next visit.

SLEEP APNEA AND SURGERY:
A DANGEROUS COMBINATION

Just recently I met with a new patient, Simon, a talented cabinet maker in his mid- to late 50s who was currently unemployed due to needing hip replacement surgery after so many years of standing. Simon had never been diagnosed with a sleep disorder, nor did he have high blood pressure. But in his presurgical evaluation, the internist (who had heard me lecture before about the higher risk of poorer surgical outcomes associated with untreated sleep apnea) noticed Simon's neck circumference measured larger than normal, the back of his throat looked narrow, and he was overweight. He suggested that Simon get checked for sleep apnea before surgery.

And so one week before his scheduled surgery, Simon arrived at my clinic for evaluation. Guess what? We discovered 100 breathing pauses per hour! (Normal is less than 5.) Also, his oxygen was dropping into the 70 percent range at night. This was a severe case of sleep apnea, and it would be dangerous to move forward with the surgery. I had to sit Simon down immediately and break the news: "I'm so sorry, but you cannot have surgery next week." Here I was canceling his surgery due to a condition he didn't even believe he had!

But here's the problem: We now know that untreated sleep apnea can lead to all kinds of dangers postsurgery. Surgery is a stress on your body, which means you're going to produce more adrenaline. Untreated sleep apnea also causes higher levels of adrenaline in the body, which increases blood sugar and is bad for the heart. That's a lot of adrenaline—which leads to poor wound healing, rising blood sugars, strain on the heart, and potentially dangerous heart arrhythmias. You are also given a big concoction of meds postsurgery (pain meds, muscle relaxers, sleep aids)—all of which make sleep apnea even worse.

Surgery is a firestorm for the body, no matter how small that surgery is, and untreated sleep apnea is like pouring gasoline on the fire. Or you can think of sleep apnea like a big pot of hot oil—surgery is the onions you throw into it. Just make sure to stand back; there's going to be a big splash!

I called Simon's surgeon, who agreed with my assessment. We delayed the hip replacement by three weeks so we could get him started on CPAP and get this problem under control. I can say with confidence this intervention saved his life (had he gone on to have the surgery untreated), and we increased his longevity too. Simon has a new hip now—in addition to a better life and most likely fewer heart problems in his future.

PART III:

WHAT DOES BETTER SLEEP LOOK LIKE?

Chapter 8

While You Were Sleeping...
during the Pandemic

*Sleep Vigilanteism: Like so many of life's other
fortunes—health, youth, success, happiness—
sleep is not valued till it's gone.*

Those of us who lived through March 11, 2020, will never
forget that on this day the world changed: The World
Health Organization declared COVID-19 a pandemic. We will
now forever view life in terms of the "before times" and the
"after times."

As both an internist and a sleep physician, I watched this
all unfold from the unique perspective of both fields. Due
to my medical training, background, and the hospital staff
shortages, I worked the front lines, not only taking care of my
own patients (many of whom tested positive), but also working in the hospital on weekends, helping my partners take
care of many active COVID patients admitted to the medical
ward. When I wasn't lost in those difficult moments, I found

respite in my clinic office, helping patients with their sleep, or with family.

It's sometimes hard to believe it's been almost two years since then (as I'm writing this chapter, anyway). Back in the early days of the pandemic, every night I'd go to sleep only to wake up to some new, distressing headline—each one worse than the last. But it wasn't just me: We were all imprisoned inside this nightmare together, and we couldn't break free.

Before long, something extraordinary became apparent, and it kind of surprised me: Humanity's sleep—collectively, globally, as a whole—was collapsing under the weight of this pandemic, and it was affecting *all* of us, everywhere, together, for the first time . . . ever. The stress of our new normal was changing sleep across the board—even mine! It seemed no one was immune. The Sleep Vigilante, who keeps a close eye on sleep highs and lows every single night, never imagined he'd see something so disruptive in his lifetime.

This pandemic—the biggest global medical event for our generation—was something everybody could relate to. You just had to be human to experience it. Every person's sleep was affected. Every aspect of humanity was taken to the cleaners. You learned what was important to you and what was not. Health suddenly felt even more imperative than it did before. If you were in good health, you hoped your immune system would protect you from becoming a statistic. And if you didn't have a good support structure and smiles around you, your misery factor quadrupled.

Even the news headlines reflected this trend, coupled with this insatiable need for information about sleep, immunity, and dreams. And right away, the busy journalists came calling. Since early 2020, I have been interviewed on TV and in dozens of news articles about sleep for major media outlets, including the *Washington Post*, Martha Stewart, CNET, *Parade*, and MSN. With the pandemic in full swing, I found myself providing interviews almost weekly, and friends of mine were recognizing my name in the news. Never before had I seen such widespread, global interest in sleep health! Everyone wanted to know, Why am I having nightmares? Why are my dreams so vivid right now? Why is my insomnia so bad? Can sleep help our bodies fight the coronavirus? And on and on.

What exactly was going on with our sleep, anyway? I've thought about this a lot, and it occurred to me that just like with a human pregnancy, our relationship with sleep during the first nine months of the pandemic can be broken up into three distinct sections, or trimesters. During each of these trimesters, many of us experienced similar thoughts, stressors, feelings, and impacts regarding our sleep. See if any of the following feel familiar to you.

The First Trimester: March–May 2020

The year 2020 started out great, didn't it? We got to be excited, hopeful, and optimistic for a sparkly new year—for a couple of weeks, anyway, until we read foreboding news of a cruise ship passenger testing positive for COVID in the United States. It was unsettling, but we didn't yet know how difficult and life altering this disease was going to get.

The pandemic was an unexpected event for a lot of people (though probably not for virologists or epidemiologists). And then in March, just like a quick drugstore test that says,

"Surprise, you're pregnant!" the WHO told us, "Surprise, we're in a pandemic!"

In the first trimester of a pregnancy, your life changes drastically. It's too early to feel the joy of the baby kicking. The mother usually feels nauseated and ill a lot of the time. And so were we, in a sense, during the first months of the pandemic: We faced job losses. Lockdowns. People losing income. Loneliness. Panicked toilet-paper buying. Upcoming summer vacations canceled. Kids in Zoom school driving everyone crazy at home. We were fearful and miserable and gaining weight.

When something unexpected happens in your life (especially if it's negative), it can be a triggering event that causes stress. And what does stress cause? Sleep problems. As a direct result of the pandemic, we began to witness a "leftward shift" of the sleep needle: Great sleepers who usually logged an easy eight hours now slept well (but not great). Good sleepers started experiencing average sleep. Poor sleepers prior to the pandemic—well, now they hardly slept at all. They fell into a really bad pattern of lost and broken sleep. (And for some, it continues to this day.) The leftward shift meant we were *all* sleeping a little or a lot worse now than before.

The Leftward Shift

The stress of the pandemic made everyone's sleep a little bit worse:

Worst Sleepers ← Worse ← Poor ←
Average ← Good ← Great Sleepers

The Second Trimester: June–August 2020

I think a lot of us started getting used to things by the summer. The vaccine trials were coming. People started sleeping at home more, sleeping in, and dreaming more. Executives used to jetting across time zones were stuck at home with empty calendars and suitcases pushed to the back of a closet. For a lot of the working population used to toiling in offices, schedules shifted from commuting on freeways to shuffling from bed to desk in pajamas and fuzzy slippers.

Frazzled parents hadn't rushed to plop their kid on a 7:30 a.m. school bus for months. They were settling into the homeschooling routine. Baking bread. Peloton-ing. Kids were getting up later too, and the mood of the household started improving. This is just like how things get better during the second trimester of the pregnancy: People are complimenting her now on her pregnancy glow; the nausea isn't as bad; she's sleeping great. The first summer of the pandemic stands out because so many of us recaptured the lost sleep and vibrant dreams we had been missing out on for a long time. A lot of us got used to the luxury of sleeping later. We rediscovered the kind of effortless, healing sleep that had evaded us for far too long in our prepandemic lives. I saw this in my patients, my family, my friends, and even myself. If there were ever a silver lining to this pandemic, this was it.

I understand that frontline health care workers, those in service industries, and others experiencing higher levels of stress (like being unable to pay their bills, getting sick, or knowing people who died) didn't experience this luxury. Their sleep changed, too, but unfortunately for the worse.

The Third Trimester: September–November 2020

In the third trimester of a pregnancy, anxiety levels heighten. There's nervousness and uncertainty surrounding the impending delivery; the parents rush to get the nursery in order; the reflux burns worse than before. As if that wasn't bad enough, the pregnant woman gets so swollen and uncomfortable that she can't sleep well anymore (not to mention all those late-night bathroom breaks!).

By this time in the pandemic, a lot of people started going back to work again (in masks this time), even though a lot would have preferred to keep working from home. Fear and stress levels skyrocketed, death tolls spiked, people were losing loved ones (or knew someone who did), the vaccine data results weren't in yet, and we had all the drama surrounding the election.

We also saw a rise in "revenge bedtime procrastination," when people willingly put off their sleep to do something else even though they know they'll feel terrible tomorrow. The days started blurring together, and more of us reached for the remote instead of the pillow just so we could binge-watch the latest addicting series late into the night (to subsequent regrets in the morning). At the same time, a lot of people started misusing sleep medications. They had more nightmares than before. We'd endured the stress for too long and were coping in unhealthy ways. And things didn't seem to be getting any easier.

We had also lost our important circadian cues that come from getting out into the world, which guided us so much in our prepandemic lives. So now we missed:

- **social cues** by not meeting up with friends like we used to,
- **light cues** from being sedentary and sitting indoors all day and binge-watching favorite shows and social media channels late into the night, and
- **food cues** by eating delivery instead of in restaurants or dining rooms with loved ones and snacking all the time.

These vital sleep-wake signals work in harmony to ensure healthy sleep, and when we lose sight of them, our sleep gets mixed up too. When restaurants, malls, offices, schools, and borders closed and people went into lockdown all over the planet, they didn't realize how important these little daily signals would be to retaining their healthy sleep rhythm long term (not to mention their mental health).

I actually created an acronym to explain how a lot of us felt at this time. We were **FED UP** (and many of us still are), which stands for the following:

Financial stress
Emotional stress
Distance from others
Unpredictability
Personal and professional stressors

And so our sleep suffered. When you are that FED UP, how could it not?

By this time, December loomed. If all goes well, a healthy pregnancy ends after nine months, leaving the new mom and dad with a cute, cranky baby that probably bawls with clenched fists all night. After nine months of the pandemic, we weren't so lucky—but we did get something else entirely different.

Congratulations! We Birthed a New Sleep Disorder

It isn't often a new term enters the sleep lexicon. It also isn't usual that we slog through a never-ending, Earth-circling pandemic. But that's what the 2020 stork brought us. And so here we are.

You've probably heard of "coronasomnia" by now (and maybe even experienced it). The sleep problem, a clever combination of the words *corona* and *insomnia*, has become quite common in my clinic since mid-2020 and is so widespread now that even my friends and family have reached out for advice, tips, and suggestions on what to do.

> **Coronasomnia:** Insomnia caused by the stress, anxiety, and poor sleep habits brought on by the coronavirus pandemic

It's interesting to note here that coronasomnia is an epidemic inside of a pandemic—a "tandemic." Prior to 2020, chronic sleep loss was already an issue, a "public health problem" according to the CDC. But the pandemic's leftward shift I described earlier has pushed even *more* people into troubled sleep, making an already bad situation even worse.

So what does coronasomnia look like in the average person? I'm going to share some interesting patient case studies for you here, along with the successful techniques we used to combat it. Keep in mind, the first two examples are people who *didn't* have COVID. After that, you'll meet someone who did, and you'll learn about the debilitating sleeplessness that so often lingers in long-haulers post–COVID infection and what we did to help her.

Case Study #1: Justin, a 30-Something Video Editor for a Professional Sports Team

Justin has this amazing but demanding job working as a video editor for a professional sports team. But back when the pandemic hit, he found out his job wasn't as stable as he thought. He worked for a different team at the time, and that position was going fine until the lockdowns happened. Then just like that, he was let go like so many others.

Now he found himself home all the time, jobless. That is a huge, stressful event even by itself—but now factor in the pandemic. He lost his daily structure, his socialization, his work responsibilities, his healthy sleep habit of 11 p.m. to 6 a.m., his daily workout, and so much more. He was struggling and unable to find work, and before long he started eating meals at weird hours of the day, sleeping poorly, and feeling depressed and anxious. His doctor prescribed sleeping pills, but when he came to see me, he said he didn't want to take them anymore. Plus, they weren't even helping anyway.

Fast-forward several months. Justin finally found work with a new team—an excellent development for his self-esteem, career, and sense of purpose—but unfortunately, the poor sleep habits were cemented at this point. Now he had a great job but not-so-great sleep. He found himself sleeping well four days a week but then would lie awake and ruminate with terrible insomnia the other three. He was really only sleeping half the time—no wonder he felt awful!

Because insomnia (and especially coronasomnia) is so often psychological, my prescription for Justin involved important behavioral changes with the expectation that he could drop his sleep meds soon. First, I asked him to manage his light exposures and try not to stare into bright screens so close to bedtime—a suggestion that admittedly would be a little bit hard for him to implement, considering his line of work. The games don't even end until 10 p.m., and then he's often up late doing postgame media, chopping replays for the coaches, and so on.

I also asked him to find a healthy way to unwind from the day and create a relaxing bedtime structure using my Four-Play Method. (See chapter 10 for details on how you can make this work for you too.) Grateful for the guidance on how to fix his sleep, Justin agreed to try everything.

Justin is still a new case for me, but I know he'll get his sleep under control and be feeling great again soon. He was already feeling better after just a few days of my methods—which is so important for the buy-in of my (or any) sleep program. A few days of quality sleep can really motivate you not only to make the necessary lifestyle changes but also to help you feel confident that you can experience peaceful nights of quality sleep again and again.

Case Study #2: Brooke, a 46-Year-Old Scientist

Brooke, a scientist for a large pharmaceutical and research corporation, first came to see me for her terrible insomnia four years ago. Hers was very much a classic case: She had a family history of the common sleep disorder, but it didn't get triggered in her own life until she experienced a major stressor, which was a breast cancer diagnosis and the subsequent treatment for it. After introducing cognitive behavioral therapies for her to follow and working to reduce the hyperactivity of her mind in the evenings, we were able to wean her off her sedative medication and teach her to experience restful sleep once again.

I didn't see her again until the pandemic hit. Her insomnia, managed for so long, went rogue and wrecked her sleep just like before. Looking closer, I saw that not only was she FED UP, but she had also lost those little circadian cues (social, light, and meal times) that we all rely on throughout the day to keep our sleep rhythm in check. No longer in a busy office, she now worked remotely 100 percent of the time in her home and spent long hours on the computer. Like so many of us, she lost her daily structure, adopted a sedentary lifestyle, and took in way too much screen exposure. Pile onto that the uncertainties and anxieties surrounding the pandemic, plus her innate tendency for insomnia, and you have the makings of a coronasomnia disaster!

The good news is she didn't wait too long to see me. (The longer insomnia goes unchecked, the harder it is to treat.) I asked her to

- add structure to her routine again,
- manage her light exposures,
- schedule meals at the proper times,
- make it a priority to leave the house every day,
- stop working at a decent hour in the evening,

- exercise every day, and
- take a prescription sedative in the short term.

It really isn't hard to do these things, but it does require discipline, which can be difficult when you are exhausted from sleepless nights and feeling unmotivated. But once you experience a few good nights of sleep, it gets easier to follow the plan.

Like training wheels, the prescription medications were used while we worked to enhance her natural sleep drive and eliminate the obstacles. It didn't take long for her to regain her balance and learn how to ride the "sleep bicycle" again—all along knowing that her ultimate goal would be to drop the meds and sleep on her own with confidence.

Case Study #3: Seema, an Active Runner in Her 50s (and COVID Long-Hauler)

In December 2020, before the vaccines received emergency use authorization, Seema woke up one morning feeling terrible. Her throat burned. She had a high fever and body shivers. She lost her senses of taste and smell and started to cough and have trouble breathing. She went to her doctor for a PCR test and soon got the result: COVID positive.

Prior to this, Seema was an active and healthy 50-something who loved to run in her spare time. COVID took that away from her for several months. But it stole something else from her too: her sleep.

No one sleeps well when they are ill, and COVID sufferers are no different. But even as they begin to heal from the virus, and they start to feel a little bit better than before, an uncomfortable cough so often lingers for longer. Seema found this to be the case: She would wake up with night sweats, breathless and coughing, and then have trouble falling back asleep. This pattern continued to interrupt her sleep night after night for several months. Frustrated and in discomfort, Seema didn't want to just lie there in her bed and stare at a dark ceiling. And so she started getting up at 3 a.m. and doing other things. Folding laundry. Emptying the dishwasher. Doing other chores. And then eventually, she'd come back to bed even more exhausted than before.

It took a long time, but her cough did heal. Her insomnia, however, remained. Because even when the coughing stops, the unhealthy sleep patterns that were repeated over and over persist. These perpetuating behaviors make up the third *P* of insomnia, which I talked about earlier in this book. (The first *P* is genetic predisposition; the second *P* is precipitating factor.) Once formed, these habits must be broken.

It's a hard road with COVID long-haulers. There's still so much we don't know about this disease, and it's difficult to keep up when the virus continues to mutate. It's challenging to formulate a single solution for everyone; there is this whole variation of infection in people, and people respond differently to the virus. In many cases, we are learning as we go. We do know that sleep disorders have emerged from pandemics before, and now that we are going through one again, we want to keep our eyes open. We also know that historically, we see more sleepiness and neurological symptoms like brain fog in people in the aftermath of viral infections, and COVID is no exception.[1] One 2021 study found that those who tested positive for COVID-19 had three times the risk of sleeping problems.[2] Your sleep-wake rhythm is controlled by important brain mechanisms, and research shows that COVID harms the brain. Studies have also shown that patients with obstructive sleep apnea are at greater risk: One 2020 study showed they were eight times more likely to get COVID compared to others in their age group.[3]

For Seema, who luckily had begun to heal from her coughing, I took a traditional approach to her treatment. I still remember ripping off a large piece of butcher paper in my office and drawing out my "Cot of Dreams" plan for her (Fig. 81). For me, it really adds that personal touch for the patient. They feel more invested when I sketch out their plan in permanent marker, and I believe it also helps them visualize and retain their next steps.

And so I asked Seema to

- follow my Four-Play Method in chapter 10,
- improve her sleep drive during the day using the various strategies discussed in this book,
- lower her stress levels, and
- turn her clock away from the bed.

Turning your clock away from your line of sight is so important! It's tempting to want to check the time when you can't sleep, but doing so just works you up with a "doomsday countdown." This happens when you look at the clock and say, "OK, it's 4:25 a.m. If I fall asleep right now, I still have exactly two hours and five minutes to sleep until my alarm goes off." We all sometimes do this (even me!), but you must resist the urge. Nothing good comes from it. (It's even worse

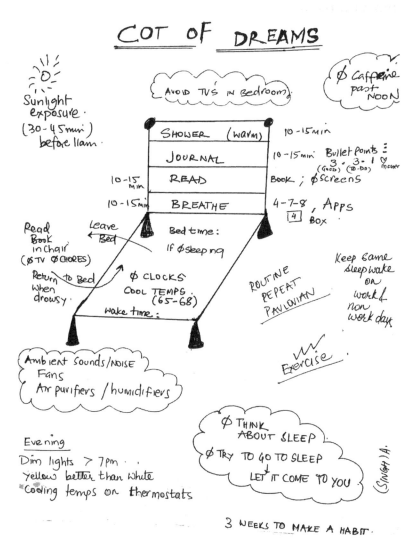

FIGURE 8.1. My "Cot of Dreams" visual, tailored to each patient, helps them reflect, understand, and truly embrace their new plan for better-quality sleep.

for a sleep physician. I'm not only doing arithmetic; I'm also dividing my sleep cycles by thirds to try to calculate how much REM I can still get!)

Sleeping well is very much dependent on discipline—having the willpower to follow a healthy sleep routine, to set up the right environment, and to curb activities that may feel good right now but actually harm your sleep. Luckily, once patients experience one good night of quality sleep, then two . . . their confidence renews, and they believe they can achieve more. They learn that their bad sleep is not a dead end. One year since her COVID diagnosis, I'm happy to report that Seema committed to the plan, was able to drop the sleep sedatives prescribed by her doctor, and now sleeps as well as she did pre-COVID.

The other thing Seema did right was to get help for her insomnia *before* it morphed into what I call an "insomnia cactus." The insomnia cactus grows big and strong when you get really good at not sleeping well. It sets down roots, and then the spiny, paddle-shaped stem of insomnia pushes up through the earth. You don't even have to water it now for it to live at this point, and you definitely don't want to touch it! Once the insomnia cactus sprouts and takes shape, the thing grows on autopilot. Your terrible sleep patterns now have a life-force of their own and are much harder to tame.

I use my "Cot of Dreams" sketch mentioned earlier to make sure my patients pay attention. I don't ever want them to get "good" at not sleeping well. When I can prevent insomnia from happening—from growing into a full-blown cactus—it feels like a save. And it's one of the most rewarding aspects of my job.

The Sleep-Immunity Connection

People usually don't think about this, but sleep is essential for the daily servicing of your immune system.[4] For obvious reasons, this matters every single day when you encounter germs and other viruses in your environment. But also think back to the first year of the pandemic, when we didn't have vaccines yet. What did we have to protect us? The only thing we had was our immune systems. Especially in the first days and weeks of this new, unprecedented virus infecting host victims exponentially: We didn't have any defenses whatsoever. Whoever had the strongest immune system won.

We know that sleep loss means a four-times higher risk of developing the common cold.[5] Sleep loss also means poorer wound healing. Even vaccines rely on your immune system to create immunity, and research has shown they function better when you get plenty of quality sleep before and after inoculation. That all tells you something: Sleep has always been your hidden antidote before any antidote was discovered. And that goes for any illness, especially viral illnesses. How wonderful that sleep reconditions and services your immune system every night.

If we could peek inside our bodies while we slept (and I'm talking quantity *and* quality sleep here), we would see that during the first half of our sleep, our bodies generate pro-inflammatory cytokines. Cytokines are tiny proteins, or peptides, that serve to regulate inflammation, immune response, and hematopoiesis. (Hematopoiesis is the production of blood cells, including T cells, which are white blood cells that fight infections.)

Cytokines are angry, little aggressive molecules that go and kill stuff. They attack the germs and whatever else doesn't look right. Your immune system knows to make more of them when you are sick—and all those extra cytokines running around activate your sleep drive, making you feel tired when you are fighting something. You can also think of them as tiny hedge cutters that trim back all the wild branches and greenery encroaching on your house.

But who is going to clean up all the clippings left behind? That's why the second half of your sleep is so important. This crucial time is when lots of anti-inflammatory chemicals sweep through and clean up the mess left by the cytokines. They power wash everything away and refresh your body for another day. But when you fail to get enough sleep, or you chop your sleep off halfway through, this elegant process of cleaning up germs gets interrupted and fails to complete. The mess doesn't get cleaned up properly, and now you're starting your day like that.

My hope is that you will learn to love sleep, which is why I've made that the focus of my next chapter. So many people willingly put off sleep without fully understanding the impacts of that decision. Or you disregard seeing a sleep physician because you think you've adapted to living with terrible sleep. (*Note:* You haven't.) This is especially important now, in these "after times": If you or a loved one is a COVID long-hauler dealing with protracted symptoms, I strongly encourage you to get evaluated for a sleep disorder. It just may be the missing piece to your healing puzzle.

The next time you stay up extra late to scroll social media reels, watch one more episode, fold laundry at odd hours, or read one more chapter with half-lidded eyes, remember that your immune system would really like that sleep you're neglecting. (Let's make sleep go viral!)

Chapter 9

Fall in Love with Sleep Again

Sleep Vigilanteism: Like a soulmate, your perfect sleep is out there somewhere. Are you ready to let it find you?

Most people love sleep, or at least the idea of it. Cozy mornings while on vacation. Waking up from a beautiful dream that feels almost too real. Feeling completely rested upon awakening, even before you brew that first cup of joe or tea.

The reality of sleep, however, doesn't always live up to expectations. In fact, all too often it doesn't even come close. If it did, we wouldn't need sleep researchers, sleep scientists, or sleep physicians like me. I would be out of work with no patients, and you'd probably find me following a completely different path in life. I'd be an educator of some sort, or perhaps a music producer. For me, everything in life is about finding rhythm, whether I'm making music in my spare time or following brain and breathing patterns on a polysomnogram.

In our modern, fast-paced, screen-focused world, far too many of us have ended up disconnected from this natural, gentle, and healing process called sleep. Sleep is supposed to be intuitive, but sleep takes time—time we just don't have (or think we don't have). When you run yourself ragged with work commitments, your social life, and the new streaming series that can't wait, sleep doesn't quite fit in. And so it gets pushed to the side more frequently than you'd care to admit. Eventually, you toss and turn most nights and forget that you used to like sleep at all. And there's probably a comforting bottle of sleeping pills rolling around in your nightstand.

When I work with patients on improving their sleep, a big part of what I'm asking them to do is to prioritize sleep in their daily lives. That usually means behavioral modifications in addition to carving out time for sleep. I ask them (and now you) to set aside approximately *one full hour* every night for my Four-Play Method, which you'll learn about in the next chapter. This isn't a one-night stand we're talking about—it's a commitment to sleep that I hope lasts a lifetime.

This kind of change is easier to embrace when you love something. Love inspires you to do better. When you love something (and remember, love is an "action" word),

- you make it a priority,
- you make sacrifices for it,
- you look forward to it,
- you crave it,
- you make time for it,
- it feels easy,
- it brings out your best,
- it makes you smile, and
- it makes you glow.

So many patients I see have already fallen out of love with sleep. They don't like it; they don't look forward to it; it doesn't feel good; they dread it. Maybe they're terrible sleepers; maybe they struggle with insomnia; maybe their spouses snore like freight trains. They've developed negative associations that feel irrefutable and ingrained. They sleep poorly or feel tired all the time and have gotten used to this low bar as their "new normal." That's where I come in, to help them get back to where they once were. Because this is not a place they want to be: They want to reconnect with the kind of great sleep they remember having once upon a time.

Everyone can improve their relationship with sleep, no matter their situation, challenges, or level of doubt. (See "Top Five Sleep Disorders" on the next page.) Whatever it is right now, you can make it better. Even if you think you sleep great, you can (and should) take it up a notch so you can protect what you have even during tough times. Every one of us has the potential inside to learn to love (or at least really like) sleep again.

Removing Barriers to Sleep

Teaching people how to love sleep again is so important for so many reasons, as outlined in this book already—not to mention the very basic reality that being alive means sleeping every single night. You are bound to sleep for a lifetime; you might as well get good at it!

For people with a history of unhealthy patterns related to sleep, reframing these anxieties and negative experiences as solvable and offering reliable solutions can help. For those plagued by a sleep disorder, identifying the issue (and working through it) finally provides the relief sought for so long.

The secret is, once the problem sleeper experiences one luxurious night of sleep, and then another, the ensuing domino effect inspires them to reach for (and achieve) more.

Top Five Sleep Disorders

1. Behaviorally induced (self-inflicted) sleep deprivation, where you don't give yourself adequate opportunities to sleep
2. Insomnia
3. Snoring/sleep apnea
4. Restless legs syndrome
5. Narcolepsy and circadian rhythm problems

Note: This list is my personal perspective, based on my years as a clinician.

When you've had the fortune of helping more than 7,000 patients like I have, recurring refrains, myths (which are covered later in the chapter), and excuses regarding sleep get told to you over the years. All too often, these misperceptions impede a person's ability to sleep well. While deeply held beliefs about sleep can be difficult to change, it's not impossible. I have seen it firsthand many times: Once people learn how to nourish their relationship with sleep, sleep flourishes.

Here's a closer look at how I've helped numerous patients reframe their various sleep constructs over the years so they could go on to achieve their best sleep. Just imagine for a moment: A patient walks into my office, sits down, and says, "But Dr. Singh . . ."

PROBLEM #1: "I DO EMBARRASSING THINGS IN MY SLEEP."
My job is to show them they don't have to live like this, and we absolutely can help them. One of my most interesting cases to date was that of 66-year-old Walter, a kind soul who suffered from a curious and uncomfortable case of nocturnal eructation (nighttime belching) in his sleep. The case was so fascinating and unprecedented, in fact, that it did not yet exist in medical literature. And so I coauthored a paper on my findings.*

His wife explained to me that every night, Walter would seem to be sleeping peacefully, but then he'd start gasping for air and experience extremely disruptive eructation events in the bed all night long. It was so unpleasant, she had to sleep in another room. This didn't happen during the day, she assured me—it only happened at night. He'd tried everything before coming to see me: propping his head up on pillows, sleeping sitting up, taking antibiotics and a course of metoclopramide (typically used to increase gut motility), trying proton pump inhibitors (typically used to treat acid reflux and GERD, or gastroesophageal reflux disease), getting an ultrasound of his gallbladder, doing an endoscopy, and more. But nothing helped, and no one could solve this mystery.

---

* Abhinav Singh et al., "Nocto-Crypto-Eructo: A Rare Case of Persistent Nocturnal Eructation Treated with PAP Therapy for Obstructive Sleep Apnea: A Case Report," *Annals of Sleep Medicine* 3 (May 5, 2021), https://doi.org/10.36959/532/323.

Because he had a history of snoring and reported daytime sleepiness, we performed an overnight polysomnogram, which showed moderate obstructive sleep apnea. We started him on CPAP therapy that very night, and within four weeks, he (and his wife) reported 100 percent resolution of his nighttime burping problem. His symptoms remain resolved to this day, and he remains compliant with therapy and checks in once a year to see me with a smile on his face.

Imagine how Walter would have suffered for the rest of his life had he not followed through on getting the sleep study. But now he can look forward to sleeping and not worry about bothering his wife. So many people don't realize that it's an actual sleep disorder wreaking havoc on their sleep—and their life. This case study also illustrates how sleep apnea sometimes presents in unusual ways, and so we must be extra alert to it.

In another one of my patients, severe sleep apnea (left untreated because he could not tolerate his CPAP) caused him to engage in violent dream enactments while sleeping. This was not only embarrassing to Luke; it was dangerous. This 40-year-old handyman woke up with holes in the drywall and bruises and scratches on his face. Sometimes he unknowingly hit his wife in his sleep! He was so deprived of quality sleep that he lost his job, he was sleeping in a separate room, and his marriage was hanging by a thread. Luke was so tired he could barely hold his eyes open when he slumped over to snooze in the chair in my office.

I was so glad he overcame his fears of acknowledging this behavior and came to see me. We reduced the episodes tremendously by finding the right sleep apnea treatment: a bilevel PAP with higher pressures. Before long, he was happy, working, and sleeping with his wife again in the same bed.

Let these stories serve as a comforting reminder that you don't need to be embarrassed about a particular sleep problem. Your physician has seen it all and can help you.

PROBLEM #2: "I DON'T WANT TO USE A CPAP OR BILEVEL PAP. IT'S NOT SEXY."

I can't tell you how many times I've heard the younger men diagnosed with sleep apnea share this sentiment with me. They sleep horribly and experience fatigue and sleepiness during the day but feel strongly that using a CPAP interface to sleep at night is going to make them look completely unsexy to their partner. I understand what they are saying, but they're kind of missing the point: You know what's really unsexy? Not treating your sleep disorder. Research shows that ignoring a sleep apnea problem means less testosterone, a lower sex drive, sexual performance problems, erectile dysfunction, less sexual satisfaction, and a decrease in intimacy. I promise you, you and your partner will *love* your CPAP therapy if things sizzle (instead of fizzle) in the bedroom. And that goes for men and women.

PROBLEM #3: "CPAPS ARE BULKY AND UNCOMFORTABLE. MAYBE I DON'T NEED ONE."

If you have sleep apnea, yes, you do need to treat it! There is this prevalent belief out there that CPAPs are bulky and noisy. Patients tell me, "No, I just can't handle it." The great thing about CPAPs is they've been around 40 years. Today, there are more than 150 variations and interfaces to choose from!

We don't even call them masks anymore. They're like jeans: Walk into a jeans store and pick out what you want. Or you can think of sleep interfaces like couture shoes and purses (as my mentor Dr. Lisa Wolfe, a pulmonary and sleep medicine doctor at Northwestern, so brilliantly put it): Every fall and spring, there's a new line. With the help of your doctor, you will find the right one for you. Once you give it a try and get it working for you, you will experience higher-quality sleep at night, feel so much better in the daytime, and wonder why you waited so long to sleep this great.

I really like to underscore for my patients that the technology available now to treat sleep apnea is much different than what you are thinking in your mind. Pop culture probably dropped an image in your head, but keep in mind that usually runs about 10–15 years behind the science. And you may not even need a CPAP: Other strategies for treating sleep apnea include mouth appliances, posture devices, and nasal passage improvements (via surgery or medications), depending on the patient. The best course of action is to meet with your doctor.

PROBLEM #4: "I DON'T HAVE A SLEEP PROBLEM."

Denial is probably my favorite misperception from people who obviously aren't sleeping well, and I'm telling you I have encountered it hundreds of times. It even led me to develop my not-so-scientific (yet) triple Singh Sign test. The following test is so accurate, in fact, that if the patient sitting in front of me checks all three of the following boxes, then I know he or she *definitely* has a sleep disorder and successful treatment awaits:

- Singh Sign 1: He or she says, "Oh, I'm fine. I'm just here because of my spouse."
- Singh Sign 2: The spouse has also come to the appointment.
- Singh Sign 3: The spouse has filled out all the paper work, with the actual patient wondering why he or she is here.

Here's an example of what happens next: the spouse says the patient snores, but the patient disagrees or says it's not that bad. But because all three of the Singh Signs are present, I conduct a sleep study on the patient and confirm a sleep apnea diagnosis. Next, I fully expect the patient to undergo treatment and be successful because he or she has the support and encouragement of the spouse (who, by the way, now loves bedtime again, with the added bonus of probably adding a few years to their partner's life).

PROBLEM #5: "MY SLEEP TRACKER SAYS I'M NOT GETTING DEEP SLEEP. HELP! I'M GOING TO GET DEMENTIA."

Although the trackers are helpful in many ways, they are not quite there yet. There's no way to know if this measurement of deep sleep is truly accurate. And yet I see a lot of sleep tracker enthusiasts who've subsequently come down with "orthosomnia," an obsession with perfect sleep that's so extreme that their worries about sleep tracker data cause them to lose sleep. (Dr. Kelly Baron, a behavioral sleep medicine specialist at the University of Utah, coined the word *orthosomnia*.)[1]

I notice this problem more in my younger patients, who grew up on technology. I like to tell them, "Do you feel refreshed after sleeping? Because if you are giving yourself the appropriate complement of hours, the brain algorithm for deep sleep will take care of itself." Nature is fully capable of deciding the correct proportion when given the chance. We don't hear people saying, "Oh, I don't think the water in my glass is wet enough."

The best aspect of a sleep tracker is that it's a *great* conversation starter about your sleep. As it stands today, a tracker may not tell you a whole lot more about your sleep than what you already know (for instance, that you're sleeping less), and it really doesn't easily change your behavior or suddenly help you start getting better sleep, does it? Nevertheless, trackers are an exciting prospect, and I talk a little more about the intersection of sleep and technology and what the future might hold in chapter 11.

PROBLEM #6: "I'VE GOT MY BLUE-BLOCKING FILTER ON. I'M GOOD NOW, RIGHT?"

Night mode and blue-light blockers can be helpful in lowering your overall light exposure, but in terms of screens, light is just one component affecting your sleep drive. Content is the other: If you're watching something exciting, scary, interesting, or violent (you get the idea), you're still ramping up your brain and reducing your sleep drive. And then there's the whole problem of digital eyestrain. I tell patients they still need to be mindful when staring at screens before bed for leisure.

PROBLEM #7: "I WAKE UP IN THE MIDDLE OF THE NIGHT, AND IT'S IMPOSSIBLE TO FALL BACK TO SLEEP."

I know it *feels* like it's impossible to fall back asleep in those difficult, dark moments. (And alas, sometimes it is.) But the more you indulge in these episodes of trying really, really hard to fall asleep, the more your sleep wheels just churn in the sand.

Next time it happens, instead of what you usually do, try this instead:

- Do not check the clock if you wake up. This is easier if you keep your phone at least five feet away from your bed.
- Try 4-5-6 breathing: Inhale for four seconds, hold for five, and breathe out for six. This adds up to 15 seconds for one breath cycle. Repeat until you hopefully fall asleep. This focused breathing exercise helps you slow things down and lean your body and mind back toward sleep.
- Stay focused on the breathing pattern. It's designed to be slow on purpose in order to anchor your mind and prevent it from drifting and attaching to random (or worrying) thoughts. Show me the genius who can actually solve a problem at 2 a.m. during a bout of insomnia!
- If that doesn't work, leave the bed, sit in a chair, and read a book. Again, do not check the time. Don't check email. Don't do chores. Don't turn the light on (except for a small reading light). If it's early enough in the night, you will start getting drowsy. At that point, get back into bed, close your eyes, and let sleep come to you.
- The next day, make sure to rev up your sleep drive using the strategies outlined in this book.

Keep in mind that working through repeating bouts of insomnia takes time. It doesn't happen in one night. It's like slowly walking into the sleep pool versus diving right in with a colossal splash. I always tell patients if they can string together a few nights of proper sleep, they'll gain more confidence, the negative associations will wither away slowly, and they will look forward to sleep again. And if your problem feels insurmountable—if it has veered into "somniphobia," or feelings of extreme dread as bedtime approaches—a physician can help you.

PROBLEM #8: "NO ONE CAN HELP ME
WITH MY SLEEPING PROBLEM."

It's true some problems are trickier than others to solve, but I always aim to find a solution that works for my patients. Mark was one of those cases: You first met him in the introduction. He is the patient of mine who slept poorly for 15 years because he couldn't tolerate the CPAP or bilevel PAP device prescribed for his severe sleep apnea. Despite multiple sleep studies, a few surgeries (to fix his deviated nasal septum and remove tissues from his nose and palate), and three sleep doctors, nothing helped. When he finally traveled across town to see me, desperate for help, I was his fourth opinion. He probably had his doubts we could help him, and the pressure was on for sure.

Luckily, I started out at an advantage because I could see *all* the strategies he'd already tried that hadn't worked. I knew the failures already and went into this knowing I'd have to try a different approach. We got to talking during my evaluation, and I learned the usual things: he still snored, struggled to sleep, suffered from sleepiness during the day and breathing pauses at night, used a nasal spray, and so on. And then he mentioned something I found incredibly interesting.

Mark mentioned he was a swimmer.

I know from working in the field for so long that swimmers tend to breathe slower than the rest of us. They tend to take longer on the exhale when breathing because they are so used to holding their breath longer. Maybe this was the key.

We went to work. I took his bilevel PAP into the advanced settings (which usually aren't used for obstructive sleep apnea) and had him lie on the exam table wearing his device. Through small manual adjustments while he took little "PAP naps," we were able to tailor it to his unique breath length. He would then take it home and try it and come back again in a couple of weeks. After three visits, we finally landed on the perfect setting. Today he's off the nasal spray, using his bilevel PAP, and loves sleeping once again.

The lesson here with sleep apnea is this: Every case is different, and sometimes a deep dive into the patient's history—in this case, discovering Mark was a swimmer—reveals exactly what's been missed all along.

How to Love *Natural* Sleep . . . (without Meds)

Part of loving sleep means knowing what sleep—*natural sleep*—feels like again. That's hard to do when you're conditioned to falling asleep with the help of a sleep aid. But just as healthy food takes time and healthy relationships take time . . . building a healthy sleep routine takes time too.

That idea feels antithetical to the "instasociety" we live in today. Everyone wants what they want, and they want it *right now*. You see the same thing with sleep problems and patients clamoring for that quick fix: Can I just pop a pill and gloss over my sleep problems, Doc? And physicians on the whole feel obligated to fix things; it's their first goal. Unfortunately, the system does not reward slower, patient, long-term strategies enough. It rewards consumerism.

In 2018, 80 percent of Americans reported struggling to sleep at least one night a week, according to *Consumer Reports*.[2] And as we learned in the previous chapter, COVID made our bad sleeping problems even worse. A 2021 survey from the American Academy of Sleep Medicine found that 56 percent of respondents reported suffering from sleep disturbances since the beginning of the pandemic.[3] Americans spent $41 billion (yes, billion!) on sleep aids in 2015, according to *Consumer Reports*, a figure expected at press time to rise to $52 billion by 2020.

Clearly, people like masking their insomnia with pills. We're not talking short term, here—they want to rely on them forever. Processed sleep is like processed food. Does it feel good? Yes. Is it good in the long run? No. Sadly, we are very much a pill-popping culture, but the uncomfortable truth is that many insomnia sufferers would get better and long-lasting results by exploring behavioral therapy recommendations under the guidance of their doctors.

Things are a little bit different in India, a contrast I noticed when I visited my family in 2021. I was having some jet lag issues myself (it takes almost an entire day to fly from Indianapolis to Delhi), so I walked into a store to try to buy some melatonin. The pharmacist looked at me like I was asking for opioids or contraband! Disgusted, he said, "That's a sleeping pill. We don't have that!"

In India, it's a cultural thing to look at sleep problems much more seriously. They don't take it lightly—they see it more as part of an anxiety or mood disorder. Here in the United States, you can find melatonin on the shelf at any pharmacy or convenience store, easy. (Plus, the clerk doesn't scoff when you buy it.) There, I had to visit four different pharmacies before anyone would sell me some. But I finally got that much-needed melatonin and was able to overcome the rest of my jet lag much more quickly with a low dose in the short term.

People take sleep aids because they work. Processed sugar also helps when you are in desperate need of food, but I don't recommend eating frosted toaster pastries with sprinkles for breakfast and dinner every single day. If you find yourself dependent on sleep aids night after night—specifically, more than three nights a week for more than three months (the clinical definition of insomnia)—then it's time to speak with your sleep physician or health care provider. Remember the "insomnia cactus" I mentioned a few pages ago? You don't want to get good at sleeping poorly. You don't want that cactus to grow and thrive. Also, you're just asking for trouble the more you deviate from nature's design by using pills.

Here's a quick rundown of some of the most popular sleep remedies I've encountered in my work with thousands of patients. Some may even be in your medicine cabinet right now.

Melatonin. Melatonin is not regulated as a prescription drug in the United States, but in some other countries, it is. When needed, I do prescribe this to my patients in small doses for short-term use due to its effectiveness and mild risk of potential side effects. As you age, the pineal gland in the brain starts to produce less melatonin, so older adults may find melatonin effective for sleep improvement. Studies on the long-term effects are limited. You can think of melatonin as the lunch bell, not the lunch. Does the lunch bell quench your hunger? No. Just because you hit it harder (i.e., take more melatonin) doesn't mean you'll feel satiated.

Prescription sedative hypnotics. There are many prescription sleep aids out there. Zolpidem (Ambien), for one, is a sedative prescribed for intermittent use and, in my opinion, is best used short term, especially during acute phases of stress. Ambien gained popularity in the 1990s because it worked great for insomnia but wasn't as habit forming as other alternatives like Valium or Xanax. But you can still become dependent on Ambien to sleep if you fail to use it as directed. (Ambien was never intended for long-term usage or to be taken in high doses.) Now that 20 years have gone by, we have witnessed some people exhibiting strange behaviors while on this drug or similar ones—such as waking up with popcorn and melted ice cream on their quilts, being found asleep in different parts of the house, and waking up with the fridge door open.

My patient Vivienne, who you may remember from this book's introduction, took temazepam (generic Restoril), another prescription sedative hypnotic, to treat her insomnia. Restoril is different from Ambien, but they are both sedatives. As Vivienne's insomnia worsened, she accidentally took higher doses of Restoril than prescribed (thinking it would help her sleep better), which in turn caused her to develop a medication-induced parasomnia: the bizarre behavior of shopping for $7,000 pairs of designer Christian Louboutin shoes online in her sleep without any memory of it. (And they weren't even in her size!) Luckily, through behavioral modifications and changes to her sedative and dosage, we were able to get her insomnia (and her bank account) back under control.

Antianxiety medications like Xanax and Klonopin also fall into this category. Controlled substances can be habit forming, and I see a lot of patients who need my help getting off of them to sleep. Either their physician does not feel they can prescribe this medication long term or the patient has read about the side effects, is motivated, and wants to stop. From Ambien to Xanax, if you need a prescription medication to sleep during a normal day without stress, then I hope to inspire you to chat with your doctor and investigate other options for managing your sleep problems.

Over-the-counter medications. Histamine blockers like Tylenol PM and Unisom are extremely popular, but I don't recommend them for long-term regular nightly use. (Especially if you are elderly, please use with caution.) The many side effects include sleepiness, dizziness, and lack of coordination. Also, tolerance can develop if used for too long.

Cannabis/THC/CBD. Now that cannabis and cannabis-derived products have become legalized in several states, some papers have been published regarding the effects of these drugs on sleep. The research is both new and mixed, but preliminary results seem to indicate these are *not* good quality sleep aids for the long term. My recommendation for now is to look elsewhere for a safer and more effective option.

Valerian root. For thousands of years, people have been using valerian as a sedative to reduce anxiety and improve sleep. Despite its history, there's not much research or data on the safety of valerian. Although some studies show most people do not experience negative side effects, others found potential side effects including upset stomach, drug interactions, headache, heart rate changes, feelings of uneasiness, and insomnia. Though rare, long-term usage can cause liver failure, so it is not recommended for people with chronic insomnia or those with liver problems.

Let meds be your last stop on your journey toward better sleep, not your first. That said, I'm a pragmatist: Everything can be used short term in my book. I'm no longer the heartless sergeant I was right after graduation. I've seen the world and learned to be a little more practical. Some sleep is better than no sleep!

But I suggest that everyone think about the long-term risks versus benefits of using pills to improve your sleep. Sleep medications are kind of like training wheels: At first, they help you learn how to ride the bike by preventing you from falling. But they do not pedal you forward and should come off at some point.

The journey has not been easy, but I can tell you that I have had success weaning my insomnia patients off their sleeping pills and teaching them how to sleep naturally again. If you find yourself frequently reaching for that bottle, it's time to speak with your physician about it. Nobody taught you how to sleep when you were a baby, and you really shouldn't have to take pills for this now.

Debunking Popular Sleep Myths

When people buy into prevailing sleep myths (for instance, "Taking a pill to sleep is no big deal!"), three things are happening. First, they are clearly not sleeping optimally. Second, they have most likely fallen out of love with sleep. Third, they are harming their health in a multitude of ways.

You can't achieve the best sleep of your life if misguided beliefs are interfering with your ability to get there. See if any of the following popular sleep misperceptions sound familiar to you. Remember, it's never too late to make changes for the better!

MYTH #1: I JUST NEED A COUPLE OF SHOTS OF WHISKEY TO SLEEP GREAT.

Reality: Alcohol does relax you, but it's terrible for sleep quality. Falling into an alcohol-induced slumber is like sleeping on a bed of thorns. The first part of that sleep feels like roses, but then the thorns poke you two hours later as you crush through the petals. On top of that, your snoring is worse, and you've got a hangover in the morning. Sleep like this enough and you just might get used to it and forget what healthy sleep is supposed to feel like.

MYTH #2: I DON'T NEED MUCH SLEEP. SIX HOURS WORKS FOR ME!

Reality: Everyone needs at least seven hours, and sometimes even eight, so they can experience all the important restorative benefits of sleep mentioned throughout this book. The later deep states especially support your memory, immune system, and more. If you're going on six hours and feeling "fine," the truth is, you've just adapted to less sleep (to the detriment of your health). You will likely end up making payments in the shape of health problems down the road on this high-interest sleep loan that you have taken out.

MYTH #3: "I'LL SLEEP WHEN I'M DEAD" (AS BON JOVI SAID).

Reality: Would you prefer to get there sooner or later? Sleep deprivation increases all-cause mortality, and untreated obstructive sleep apnea can shave 7 to 10 years off your life. Also, your quality of life as you age will suffer if you continually rack up sleep debt. Everything we know about sleep points to this: You will probably get to your fabled goal quicker if you don't sleep enough and have less years in your life and less life in your years.

MYTH #4: I'LL JUST CATCH UP ON SLEEP ON THE WEEKEND.

Reality: Unfortunately, sleep doesn't work that way. Sleep lost is sleep lost. You may remember my analogy earlier in the book about driving on a bad road filled with potholes. That's what you are doing those five nights during the week that you neglect your sleep. Even if you sleep optimally on the weekend, the damage to your car (or in this case, your body) from the previous days remains. You can't "undo" damage like that. Just do the math: If you lose two hours per night for five nights, even if you try to catch up on the weekends for two or three hours each night, you are still mathematically and (most importantly) biologically short.

MYTH #5: I'M JUST A BAD SLEEPER
GENETICALLY. IT CAN'T BE HELPED.

Reality: Everyone can learn how to improve their sleep. Even insomniacs, who come into this world with a genetic predisposition for the disorder. With the right behavioral modifications and commitment to the process, my belief is that everyone can learn how to sleep better.

MYTH #6: DAYTIME NAPS ARE BAD FOR YOU.

Reality: While it's true I believe we should relegate the word *nap* to describing what babies and toddlers do, a quick "recharge" in the early afternoon is exactly what your body and brain need to power through the rest of the day with ease. Fifteen to 20 minutes of quiet rest will help you feel brighter, sharper, and more patient.

MYTH #7: I'M A GREAT SLEEPER. I FALL ASLEEP
THE SECOND MY HEAD HITS THE PILLOW!

Reality: While this seems like a good thing to brag about, falling asleep the second you close your eyes is one of the leading signs of sleep deprivation. When you fall asleep that quickly, your body is desperately trying to tell you that you need to sleep more. My tips in the next chapter should get you back on track!

MYTH #8: I'M NOT HEAVY, SO I COULDN'T
POSSIBLY HAVE SLEEP APNEA.

Reality: We see sleep apnea in all kinds of people: men, women, thin, overweight, young, old. It's best to get checked out if you experience symptoms such as snoring, breathing interruptions, restless sleep, excessive sleepiness, and day-time fatigue. The only way to uncover this so-often "hidden" sleep disorder is to meet with a clinician and undergo a sleep study (that can also be done in the comfort of your home), which will detect if there are quantifiable breathing interruptions or pauses while you sleep.

Let's talk about sleep apnea for a moment. The interesting thing about sleep apnea patients is that they're coming to see me for something else, like what they think is mild snoring, or daytime sleepiness, or because their heart doctor wants them to see me, or because their job requires a screening for the disorder—meanwhile, they think they're sleeping just fine. Upon diagnosis (which is usually a complete surprise to them), we can institute a treatment plan that will not only improve their sleep but also hopefully address other coinciding health problems, such as reflux, dry mouth, morning headaches, daytime sleepiness, and blood pressure issues. For severe cases, long-term cardiovascular risks such as heart attacks and strokes also reduce with treatment. There's an added benefit too: Once they experience optimal sleep following treatment, they feel good, realize what they've been missing, and enjoy their sleep so much more, they can't believe they suffered from inadequate sleep for so long!

Sleep Apnea: An Arduous Journey

Getting sleep apnea patients to make changes sometimes takes some convincing. I'm going to share with you a little spiel I use to encourage them to cooperate with the treatment plan. They aren't happy about this diagnosis, but they also don't understand how dangerous it can be if left untreated. My pitch goes a little something like this.

Snoring and sleep apnea can be looked at like potholes on a road. Are they common? Yes, they are. But do you want your car to slam over them every single day? Absolutely not. If you keep hitting these potholes over and over again, you're going to damage your car. One or two here and there means your car will generally be fine. But if you keep striking them every time you drive your car, 20 or 30 of these per hour, you're going to hurt your car no matter what. It's the same thing with the human body.

Now that you've driven over hundreds or even thousands of potholes, you're going to start ordering off an appetizer menu one by one. But this is no feast you will want to partake in:

- more daytime sleepiness
- concentration issues
- memory deficits
- anxiety
- depression
- reduced quality of life
- heartburn
- reflux
- dry mouth
- relationship discord
- "ouch to couch"
- insulin resistance
- appetite dysregulation
- weight gain
- higher risk of diabetes
- sexual dysfunction
- decreased libido
- erectile dysfunction in men
- reduced immunity (a higher risk of infections; reduced responses to vaccines)

SNORE NO MORE: NOSTRIL "PILLOWS" AND THE DIDGERIDOO? BEST (SURPRISING) TECHNIQUES TO TREAT SNORING

I talk a lot about sleep apnea in this book. But just because you snore doesn't necessarily mean you need a CPAP device. Here are a few non-CPAP alternatives designed to fix your snoring problem. Just make sure to talk with your sleep doc first to find the right solution for you.

- Bongo Rx EPAP Device: Described as featuring "nasal pillows," this small device fits into your nostrils to help you breathe normally without snoring.
- eXciteOSA: This product is a "daytime therapy" that strengthens your tongue muscles to prevent snoring.
- Oral appliances: Tailor-made by your local dentist, these appliances reduce snoring by moving the lower jaw forward to create more space in the back of the throat.
- Positional therapy: Pillows are used to help a person stay on their sides while sleeping. This option targets those who only snore when on their back.
- Lifestyle changes: Losing weight, reducing alcohol before bedtime, and not smoking are all effective ways to reduce snoring.
- The didgeridoo: Learning to play wind instruments like the saxophone and the didgeridoo can

improve muscle tone in the airway and reduce
snoring. (Although I can't promise you your
partner will actually prefer the didgeridoo
over your snoring.)

- Surgery: Surgery should always be a last resort.
  Talk to your doctor about all your other
  options first.

That's just the appetizer menu. Be careful—if you don't change course right now and get treatment for your sleep apnea, you're going to continue driving over potholes. Let's say you let your moderate sleep apnea go untreated for five to seven years—now, you're ordering off the entrée section of the menu, where things get meatier and more expensive. Here are your mouthwatering (in a bad way) selections:

- higher risk of stroke, which increases with the severity of sleep apnea
- more heart irregularities (A-fib, heart blockages, an increase in cardiac events such as heart attacks in the middle of the night to 6 a.m., plus a 2.3-times-higher risk of systolic congestive heart failure)[4]
- pulmonary hypertension
- unexpected complications from surgical procedures (as you learned in chapter 7)
- sudden cardiac death

I promise you, ignoring sleep apnea is not a good deal. You are not going to love or even like ordering off this menu.

(And whatever you do, *do not ask* to see the dessert menu!) Because when sleep apnea continues without treatment, the car (your body) slowly gets damaged, and the repair bills pile up. But unlike a car, you can't trade this one in for a new one.

I hope I have encouraged my patients (and you) to please "ignore the snore no more." Your future self—and your bed partner—will love you for it!

Chapter 10

The Easy Sleep Reset

Sleep Vigilanteism: Sleep is like a butterfly. If you want to catch it, you have to let it come to you.

Imagine you have a flight to Hawaii later today. In just a few hours, you'll be exiting the plane, getting lei'd, and feeling the sand between your toes. But none of that can happen if you don't plan: First you must pack a suitcase, check in, show up an hour or two before, check your bags, and pass through security. Because we all know that if you pull up to the curb one minute before takeoff, you've missed your flight.

I often tell my patients to think of getting ready for bed as a process, much like getting ready for the airport to catch a flight is a process. The process continues once you settle in your seat: You switch your electronics to airplane mode, fasten your seat belt, and put your tray table up. Everyone follows the routine in an organized way, every single time, so the plane can enjoy a smooth takeoff. You will want to prep for sleep in much the same way, with repeating rituals, so that you can just close your eyes at pushback and drift away.

Rev Up Your Sleep Drive

Enjoying great sleep—of optimal quality and quantity—means making smart decisions throughout the day that support your circadian sleep-wake cycle. It's not as simple as what you do five minutes before you turn out the light.

The accepted model in sleep research describes the sleep-wake system as a 24-hour cycle governed by the interplay of two processes: circadian (known as process C) and homeostatic drive (process S), which perpetually interact.[1] I challenge you to think of your entire day (morning, afternoon, and evening hours) in terms of building up your homeostatic sleep drive (process S, a.k.a. "sleep pressure"), so you can feel a natural rising urge to sleep in the evening as bedtime approaches. The longer we are awake, the more the pressure builds. And when we sleep, the pressure lessens. If you tend to have problems sleeping, you'll want to make sure to build up enough sleep drive during the day. If you're not yet following something like this checklist, now is a good time to start:

Morning
- Wake up at the same time every day.
- Eat a healthy breakfast (a minimum of 12 hours since your last meal—"breaking" your fast).
- Get sunshine (15-45 minutes in the morning, no later than noon—the earlier, the better).
- Don't wear sunglasses if possible, and let that rich morning sunlight enter your eyes and help synchronize your circadian rhythm by telling your brain and body that it is "wake" time.

Afternoon
- Eat lunch (a healthy, calorie-appropriate, balanced, and nutritious lunch).
- Avoid caffeine after noon.
- Exercise.

Evening
- Eat dinner (2–3 hours before bed).
- Avoid alcohol too close to bedtime (I recommend 3 hours before bed).
- Dim lighting 2 hours before bed.
- Make your bedroom a screen-free zone.
- Don't use screens 1 hour before bed (if possible).
- Put your cell phone out of reach of your bed.
- Use cotton sheets (they keep you cool and dry).
- Use the bathroom one last time.
- Keep your room dark, cool, and quiet (approximately 64–68°F/17–20°C, or what feels cool to you; aim for 5–7 degrees lower than your usual ambient indoor temperature).
- Wear an eye mask.

Your goal is to support and nourish your circadian rhythms, whether it's day or night, so the sleep-wake orchestra can remain in a harmonious relay.

Sleep Is a Symphony

The sleep-wake cycle is a symphony that involves two important hormones: melatonin and cortisol. Melatonin can be considered the conductor of the sleep symphony; cortisol is the conductor of your wake symphony. And both need to stay out of each other's way and work cooperatively like relay runners handing the baton over to the other smoothly. When melatonin rises in response to dimming light and dipping temperatures in the evening, it promotes sleep. And at the same time, cortisol diminishes at night to allow for a smooth exchange from wake to sleep states. In the morning, as melatonin levels lessen, cortisol levels rise; therefore, we feel less sleepy and more awake. Cortisol helps increase our metabolism, heart rate, and blood pressure in a regulated way to achieve all our daytime activities. That's why in the morning, it's normal to have this rising cortisol rhythm.

This mutual exclusivity of the timing of the spiking of these rhythms is important. And that's why in the evening, minimizing the stress hormones, including cortisol, is important so melatonin can perform its important duties. Watching the news right before bed or doing an anxiety-inducing task disrupts this system and delays melatonin—often with exposure to light as well as content through screens and news media that rev up the brain. When melatonin can't initiate the sleep symphony efficiently, you're likely to become chronically sleep deprived, feel tired, and struggle through the next day.

Now that you've learned how to build up sleep pressure in the day, my next recommendation for healthy and healing sleep of proper quality and quantity (7 to 9 hours) is to use my Four-Play Method. You'll want to start it about 45 minutes to 1 hour before bedtime. (There's some flexibility here, so you can find what works best for you.)

My simple Four-Play Method, designed for long-term impact, is a lifestyle intervention founded on good habit formation. It's backed by the science of classical conditioning: how you can learn unconsciously by repeating a set of behaviors over and over again. Do them enough, and pretty soon you've developed a new behavior. (It takes three weeks of repetition for a new brain circuit to form and develop a habit.) In this case, your goal is a new bedtime routine that supports sleep onset and optimal sleep.

The Four-Play Method not only addresses the initial resolution of a sleep problem but also serves as a long-lasting guardrail to help keep you in line. You can't just follow the plan for three weeks and then go back to your old ways. For example, if you were to lose some weight after following a particular diet regimen, does that mean you can go back to old eating habits now? No.

The wonderful thing about the Four-Play Method is that everyone can benefit, whether you are unhappy with your sleep or not. Even if you think you sleep well, I encourage you each morning to ask yourself when brushing your teeth, "Did I sleep well last night?" Maybe ask someone around you for their perspective: "How did I sleep?" "Was I restless?" This is the surface I want you to start scratching. If you begin to receive feedback, don't get defensive about it. Don't just absorb it and move on with your life, which so many people tend to do. Instead, listen and do something about it. Bad sleep is like walking around with ankle weights, and after a while, it feels like your "new normal." But you can and should unlock and remove those weights. You will sleep better, feel better, and live better too.

Comprising just four steps, my Four-Play Method is deceptively simple in that it's not exactly hard to do, but the results you achieve are entirely dependent upon your commitment to the process.

I created this method eight years ago after seeing so many people early in my career struggling to sleep. Many of these people had insomnia—with varying degrees of severity. The line of sleep-deprived patients felt endless. Could there be a better way to help them?

The foundational steps in my method are things we already knew about in the sleep science community, and some of them I learned from my mentors, but I wanted to create a system of easy, memorable steps that would resonate with my patients. I selected four of the most common sleep-promoting behaviors that most people are already familiar with, figuring they'd be more likely to follow the steps that way. I didn't want to add any more inconvenience or cost to the process. This wasn't some gadget or pill; I just wanted an elegant system that was free and accessible to almost anyone. It also fulfills the first rule of medicine—"Do no harm"—which is very important to all physicians.

The responses coming in from patients who I put on my Four-Play Method were slow and reassuring. Many told me they didn't realize it would be so simple. And before long, my patients started vanishing! That's a good thing: It means they improved their sleep, gained confidence, and started not needing their annual appointments. And so I would tell them (once they went off into the sunset, no longer needing me, my therapeutic interventions, or a prescription), "Please come back anytime if needed!" And sometimes they do indeed face a setback or need guidance once again; that's just life. We all encounter unforeseen stressful events that may require extra support to conquer. You may remember Brooke from chapter 8, who managed to keep her insomnia under control on her own until the pandemic hit, and she showed up in my office again.

Think of the Four-Play Method as your structured airport ritual in preparation for your sleep flight. The process must be similar enough every night so that your body and mind can recognize it and know what comes next: "OK, now it's time for bed." If you think about it, the transition between wake and sleep is a delicate time; it's kind of like a shift change at a hospital. Shift changes are critical moments: All the nurses and doctors who are leaving the hospital have to be very careful about handing off the correct vital information to the incoming shift. They can't just jump in their cars and race off—they must protect their patients by communicating important information first. The Four-Play Method also occurs right at an important shift change, when your body is preparing to transition from awake to sleep.

Keep in mind that the Four-Play Method is not exhaustive; feel free to modify the plan to meet your own needs and create your own perfect sleep cadence as necessary.

Dr. Singh's Four-Play Method for Optimal Sleep

Step 1: Shower (15 minutes). Why a nighttime shower? Because showering gets your body ready for bed by revving up the cooling process internally. All mammals—whether nocturnal or diurnal—experience sleep onset with rapid cooling of the brain as well as core body temperatures. By taking a warm shower before bed, blood capillaries on your skin dilate, and then heat is lost more easily. This in turn helps your body's core cool down faster and supports the release of melatonin. Melatonin then signals the body to initiate the sleep process.

I also suggest my patients be mindful of using really bright lights in the bathroom so close to bedtime. Also, read through the ingredients in your shower gel. You may be surprised: Some of the popular brands put caffeine in them! You don't want to do anything that interferes with your body's natural melatonin upswing.

Step 2: Journal (15 minutes). Journaling is all about making sure you calm the "busyness" in your mind. The goal is to try to empty your mind of all the thoughts, chores, to-do lists, worries, anxieties, problems, and concerns buzzing around your brain that threaten to disrupt your sleep. You can write things down or just doodle. Think of your brain as a bucket—you want to empty the bucket onto the page so the bucket stands still when you finally snuggle in and close your eyes. Writing everything down helps release anxiety at bedtime.

Don't know where to start? You can try a commonly known organizing strategy where you write down three of your biggest highlights or achievements of the day, your one favorite moment of the day, then three things you want to achieve tomorrow (3-1-3). Doing so leaves you in a positive frame of mind right before you drift off to sleep and promotes better recall of important things you need to accomplish the next day.

Step 3: Read (15 minutes). Reading serves to steady your mind. Find something gentle or relaxing to read. A few suggestions here: Reading on paper will always be better than reading on screens (which emit light, disrupting melatonin rhythms; plus, they can strain your eyes). Also, skip that thriller or your favorite page-turner, as this kind of excitement right before bed will just make it harder to initiate sleep. Don't worry, audiobooks work well too. You can even take it to the next level and invest in a sleep mask with built-in earbuds.

Step 4: Breathe (15 minutes or less). Once you reach this crucial final step, it's kind of like letting the flight lift off and soar past the clouds so you can float into dreamland. You want to breathe slowly in and out, or perhaps even meditate—the goal is to balance your internal environment so that you have a calm mind (free of stress and worry) and a calm body (free of discomfort as much as possible). You can try 4-8 breathing—4 counts in, 8 counts out. That equals 12, or 5 to 7 breaths per minute.

Conscious breathing is an excellent way to chill your inner self. I find Indian yoga guru and philosopher Sadhguru to be inspiring when it comes to mindful breathing. He talks about how to disconnect from your worries by chanting "I am not the body" on the inhale and "I am not even the mind" on the exhale. His breathing methods are one way to help you untether yourself from the emotions and situations weighing down on you, and they fit into the Four-Play Method beautifully by not allowing your mind to bounce all over the place.

All of these activities, put together, create a calming routine that you will come to appreciate. Think of it as a runway being cleared of all the debris before a flight. Don't you just love hearing when the pilot says, "We're cleared for take-off"? You know you can finally relax now.

Just remember, don't rush. Sleep is not a swimming pool you dive into. You want to slowly wade in from the shallow end, taking your time to acclimate before you reach the depths.

Shower, journal, read, and breathe. That's it. Four easy steps.

Strapped for Time? Just 15 Minutes to Better Sleep

Maybe you're traveling, maybe you've had one of *those* days—whatever the case, if you find your day too messy and rushed to do the Four-Play Method but still desire a short wind-down that helps your body relax, spend just 15 minutes doing the following . . . and ASCEND into better-quality sleep:

Away with screens

Stretch

Cool room

Empty your thoughts into a journal

Noise (white, pink, or brown noise or other environmental sounds. White, pink, and brown noise fall on a spectrum of different auditory frequencies. White noise has a uniform amplitude across all frequencies, like a fan or TV static; pink noise favors middle to lower frequencies and is often found in nature, like wind and rain; and brown noise falls into the lower frequencies, like thunder and waterfalls.)

Dark room

Sleep Villains A to Zzz

The Sleep Vigilante knows we're not always perfect, and that's OK. But the Four-Play Method works best when also supported by behaviors and choices that reinforce your brain's internal clock. See if you can find any of these sneaky sleep villains lurking behind your back, ready to pounce and disrupt your sleep. You likely cannot banish all of them, but I encourage you to try to eliminate as many as possible, as often as possible, so you can keep that sleep runway as clear and smooth as possible. So now that you've been warned, look out for the following:

Alcohol used to bring on sleep

Binge-watching your favorite shows and social media channels late into the night

Cell phone in bed

Drifting off while still on the couch

Exercising too close to bedtime

Folding clothes at 2 a.m. because you can't sleep

Going straight to bed without unwinding

Having to go to the bathroom (drinking liquids too close to bedtime)

Indulging in a big bowl of ice cream at midnight

"Just one smoke before bed can't hurt..."

Keeping one eye on the clock when you can't sleep

Lacking a bedtime ritual

Meals too close to bedtime

Naps that exceed 20 minutes

On your laptop all day without taking breaks

Procrastinating bedtime

Quietude disrupted by environmental noise

Ruminative thinking

Screens, especially bright ones

Temperature too warm or too cold

Using weekends to catch up on sleep

Variable bedtimes and wake-ups

Working in bed

Xanax and similar medications used too often and/or in heavy
    doses

Your bed partner snoring or being restless in bed

Zzzs of improper quality or quantity (or both)

Seven Steps to Better Sleep

What if you could be sleeping better in just one week? I'm
here to tell you that it's possible and that you can start as early
as tonight. All you need to do is make one small change every
day for seven days for better sleep. Even small changes that
seem insignificant (like getting outside in the sun for a few
minutes) add up to powerful sleep game changers. If you
aren't sure where to start, try the following seven steps and
see if your patience, mood, energy, and sleep feel enhanced.

**Sunday: Let's kick off a new week with my Four-Play
Method.** The secret is in the repetition: Do this enough, and
you'll start to feel a Pavlovian response for bedtime. Commit to the method every day, and your body and mind will
learn the routine and want to stick with it.

Monday: Go to bed 15 minutes earlier than usual. Fifteen minutes doesn't sound like much, but over seven days,
that tiny change equals an extra hour and 45 minutes of sleep!

Also, we tend to focus on sleep "quality," but "quantity" is just as important (especially since the most common problem of them all is insufficient sleep, usually self-inflicted).

Tuesday: Do a quick recharge. Between noon and 2 p.m., when the circadian rhythm takes a dip, most of us tend to start feeling a little deflated. Suddenly there's that temptation to grab a doughnut or a sugary drink for a quick and dirty boost of energy. Everybody always talks about the power nap—but the reality is, not all of us can or even want to nap. The great news is, you don't have to! You can achieve the same result and get that much-needed recharge just by quieting your mind and not engaging in thought. Even just 10–15 minutes, sitting quietly with eyes closed, focusing on breathing or even meditating, is enough to feel powered up again and ready to face the rest of the day.

Wednesday: Put worry on the schedule. We all have worries—especially now with the COVID pandemic—and they always seem to disrupt our sleep, don't they? "Scheduled worry" is another habit-forming activity that will impact your sleep positively. First decide what is worrying you, then set aside 20 minutes to actively worry and think about the specific thing bothering you. (Make sure you set a time limit and be strict about it.) You can journal, take a walk, or even sit in a corner of your office. Think about your worries, evaluate them, brainstorm possible solutions. If nothing can be fixed, that's OK—at least you know you addressed them. Confronting your worries head-on earlier in the day like this means they're less likely to swirl endlessly in your mind at night. (*Note:* This does not take the place of journaling as part of the Four-Play Method.)

Thursday: Exercise smarter. Exercise is healthy, right? So it's OK to do the exercise bike at 10 p.m., yes? Unfortunately, exercising at the *wrong* time can disrupt your sleep, and this day is all about picking the best times to exercise so your circadian clock isn't thrown completely offtrack in a mistaken bid toward good health. It can be hard on those days when you leave the office late, but see if you can fit in a workout earlier in the day. (Also, you may want to go back to chapter 3, where I talked about the best times of day for coordination, reaction times, muscle strength, and so on.)

Friday: Eliminate a sleep villain. Check out my A–Zzz list of sleep villains mentioned earlier. I'm sure at least a couple on there feel a little too familiar. This day is all about banishing the one sleep villain that haunts you the most. If you're really inspired, feel free to kick out another one too. (And maybe even another.) They have no business interfering with your quest for amazing sleep.

Saturday: Soak up some sunshine. I mention this throughout the book because it is that important! Try for just 15 minutes before noon. If it's winter, and the sun seems to be in hibernation mode until Easter, you can achieve similar benefits from a light box. Grabbing this little bit of sun and/or light earlier in the day is an important factor for your internal clock.

Guess what? In just seven days, you've taken charge of your sleep routine and initiated seven mindful, impactful changes. You're learning how to synchronize your internal and external environments and how to connect with your body's natural sleep and wake signaling. You probably feel refreshed, restored, and revitalized too. Keep it up so your health, happiness, and overall well-being can radiate for all to see.

Chapter 11

Cash in Your 13.5 Million

Sleep Vigilanteism: Sleep can make the difference between whether one ages like fine whiskey . . . or yogurt.

When one person invests in healthier sleep, their world gets a little richer. If thousands or even millions of people were to improve their sleep at the same time, the impacts would be transformative and far reaching. But how do we make that happen?

Revolutions follow evolutions. Things can't change until . . . well, things change. Looking back at sleep medicine from a historical perspective, we can see that the field has already cycled through a natural evolution from art to science to commercialization.

For millennia, sleep was theoretical—no one understood it, and people held subjective beliefs about it (like we do with art). Then breakthroughs lit up laboratories, and we began to deepen our understanding of the science, and finally, businesses promoting sleep products flooded the market to try to make a quick buck. (Back in the early 2000s, we hit some turbulent commercial waters.) It's a cycle that is now circling back to the science and, eventually, back to the art once again.

What does the sleep space look like now? Critical discoveries from innovative sleep research, along with changing attitudes, are finally pushing us in the right direction: one where science reigns supreme and sleep finds its front-row seat.

A Quiet Revolution

Sleep itself is quiet, but the positives reverberate outward in infinite ways. I see this revolution as starting small and blossoming into a human chain reaction of 360 degrees that one day blankets the earth. With a course correction right now, in this generation, we can anchor primordial prevention in place for the next generation once and for all. Good sleep habits will replace bad ones and hopefully become ubiquitous. Someday, optimal sleep will be a given, just as wearing a seat belt today is a given. It will be one of public health's greatest achievements. The movement has to start sometime, somewhere. Why not tonight in your own bedroom? As derived from the "3 Cs" saying about life, take a *chance* to *choose* sleep and *change* your life.

Even though sleep science is so fascinating, if you think about it, sleep at its core is an art. You can have all the science in the world, but if you don't connect with the "art" of it, sleep will evade you. Sleep is scientific, yes, but it is an artistic endeavor too.

Think about it: Quality sleep is a feeling; it's not a number generated by a tracker, or a graph, or a score. Your heart longs for healthy sleep, and you just *know it* when you've slept well. Can you quantify how you feel after hearing your favorite song? After watching a majestic sunset? After eating a delicious meal? This is how universal the feeling of great sleep is. The science awakens us to the magic of sleep and helps us understand it better, but it doesn't necessarily get us there. Although data can empower you and shed light on the situation, only your motivation will change your behavior.

Sleep Is Wireless

You know how you power up your phone by placing it on a charging surface? You can think of your comfortable bed like a huge charging surface for your body. Simply lie down at night and wake up eight hours later ready to learn better, look better, feel better, perform smarter, feel stronger, and live better.

The Seduction of "Sleeptech"

You've probably noticed the dizzying array of sleep-promoting products hitting the market these days. You've got cooling mattresses. Pink noise machines. Brain cooling headbands. Smartwatches. Circadian reading lights. Antisnoring pillows. Climate-control beds. Aromatherapy pods with gentle music. Smart pajamas. There's even a sleep-tracking collar for dogs!

Sixty-eight percent of us have trouble sleeping at least one night a week.[1] There is a lot of desperation there for a good night's rest. And so "sleep sells." These innovative and futuristic gadgets and gizmos sound cool, but do they really help you sleep?

We're getting closer, but we haven't found any miracle cures yet. If Sleepy Juice were the answer, we'd all have fridges stocked with it. Great science takes time; like a pregnancy, you don't want to rush it. What these products do reveal is our incredible desire for better sleep. You can expect them to continue to improve as we cycle through waves of trial and error and learn even more about sleep than we do now. The demand is there, but we're still learning.

As the science becomes stronger, so will the outcomes. It is coming. Until then, we can't wait for the science to happen; we need to connect with great sleep from within, right now, this very night. We need to learn how to listen to our body's cues and get out of our own way. It's as simple as going back to the basics: Hunger equals food, thirst equals water, and feeling sleepy should equal going to sleep—*not* hitting the "next episode" button.

Maybe people reach for "sleeptech" partly because sleep doctors, clinicians, and researchers are in short supply. Very few positions open up every year, coupled with a lack of proportionate research funding. According to the National Resident Matching Program, which places applicants into residency and fellowship positions, the field of sleep medicine offered 179 positions (many of which effectively become part time because physicians often practice sleep in addition to their primary specialty) in 2021, and 12 remained unfilled. (The state of Indiana only offers one per year!) You might expect that if we were talking about a specialty that does not affect 68 percent of the population (like hand surgery, which offered 187 positions in 2021, with 7 left unfilled). By contrast, more than 1,000 cardiovascular disease positions were offered, with only 3 left unfilled. The bottom line? Despite the pervasiveness of sleep disorders in our society, most people don't think healthy sleep is cool, and sleep medicine just isn't sexy . . . yet.

DON'T "GO" TO SLEEP

Why "go" to sleep when sleep should just "come" to you? It's like a lot of things these days:

Need a cab?

Before: Stand on the corner and hail and hope.

Today: Use an app, and it comes to you.

Need money?

Before: Go to the bank and stand in line during business hours.

Today: Your money is accessible on your phone 24/7. You don't go to the bank for it; your money comes to you (PayPal, Venmo, Zelle).

Need food?

Before: Go to the restaurant and wait to be seated, wait for the food, wait for the check.

Today: Tap an order into your phone, and food arrives on your doorstep. It comes to you.

Want to watch your favorite show?

Before: Wait until it's Monday night at 8 p.m.

Today: With on-demand, you can watch whatever you want, whenever you want. The shows come to you.

It's time we changed our perceptions around "going" to sleep. Turn it around and think of sleep in a different way: as something easy to prep for that's "coming" to you. And that is the natural way it was designed in the first place.

I want to change all that. Our health and happiness will continue to suffer until we do. My hope is that you find the information, tips, and strategies in this book helpful and encouraging as you begin your journey toward improved sleep and health.

The Future Looks "Bright" . . .

Three hundred years ago, people swallowed tapeworm eggs in order to lose weight. Arsenic was used to treat syphilis. And those with lice rubbed mercury on their bodies as medicine.

We can laugh (or groan) about it now, but what will people 300 years from now say about us? Will our descendants in 2322 think we were crazy and senseless too?

Of course they will, and they'll have an infinite number of examples to choose from. But for the purposes of this book, I'll focus on this one: our blatant disregard for the three pillars of health mentioned in this book. I assure you, people in the future are going to shake their heads in disbelief and say, *What were they thinking?*

- *They gave themselves arthritis and heart attacks by just sitting and clicking and scrolling all day?*
- *They ate processed, stale, sugar-filled foods stored in plastic by the ton?*
- *They stared at bright screens till 1 a.m. and only slept a few hours a night?*
- *They sent people to the moon . . . and yet they just sat there slowly killing themselves?!*

They're going to feel mystified and perplexed because we should have known better. (Truth be told, I'm mystified and perplexed, too, out here in 2022.) We have the science, the data, the information right at our fingertips to make healthier choices . . . but we don't. We bulldoze right through our three pillars—health, nutrition, and sleep—with abandon. The difference 300 years ago was, they didn't know any better.

We can't use that excuse now. At least regarding health and nutrition. No excuses there. But sleep is still an emerging field of study. I don't believe mass enlightenment on its importance to your health, to your brain, to your immunity—see chapter 5—has truly resonated yet. We're still of the generation that grew up thinking sleep could (and should) be disregarded if you wanted to achieve great things and earn respect. Late nights were, and still are, a trophy to be won—we grew up seeing and believing this fallacy. Let us be the last generation to think this. It's reckless to continue otherwise.

Thanks to the academicians, the thought leaders, the many scientific endeavors, and the increasing numbers of sleep-deprived people taking a moment to educate themselves about the benefits of healthy sleep, I believe we're on the brink of something exciting and revolutionary.

The future of sleep looks bright . . . and when you're talking about sleep, a "bright" future isn't bright at all (after sundown, anyway). Someday people will embrace when night falls; humanity will harmonize with their natural circadian cues; we'll know to dim the lights when the stars shine and feel good doing so. We'll all sleep to heal because we'll want to feel refreshed, restored, and revitalized for a new day and a healthier day after that. It will feel antiquated to do otherwise. Because better sleep equals better health, which equals a better life.

The Sleep Vigilante dreams that one day

- every health professional will make sleep screening a part of their daily routine patient care;
- sleep (*not* sleep deprivation) will be a trophy we'll all want to win;
- each one of us will ask ourselves every morning as we look in the mirror, "Did I sleep well last night?"; and
- the night will belong to sleep only, and we will continue to choose darkness at night, not light.

And so tonight as evening closes in (as it has on this book) and you crawl into bed and switch off the light, think back to that $13.5 million sleep fund of yours I mentioned earlier. Are you ready to cash in? Our brighter future can begin tomorrow.

Sleep Lexicon

360 degrees of sleep awareness: When you share the philosophy of sleeping better to live better with anyone and everyone around you—family, friends, neighbors—to create a geometric spread of sleep awareness.

adenosine: A chemical inside the body that builds up throughout the day as you use energy. Adenosine buildup causes more and more sleep drive (a.k.a. homeostatic sleep drive).

ATP (adenosine triphosphate): Little energy packets for the cells in your body. After they are used up, adenosine is left behind.

beta-amyloid: A metabolic waste product in the brain, the accumulation of which is linked to dementia and Alzheimer's.

bilevel PAP (bilevel positive airway pressure): A therapy for patients with sleep apnea that delivers two pressures—an inhale pressure and an exhale pressure.

bruxism: Grinding your teeth while sleeping.

cerebrospinal fluid (CSF): The fluid that our brains and spinal cords bathe and float in all our lives.

circadian edge: Achieving internal and external harmony and synchrony so that you can live strong, achieve your goals, and perform at peak level.

circadian rhythm: Our internal 24-hour clock that also regulates our sleep-wake cycle.

coronasomnia: Insomnia caused by the stress, anxiety, and poor sleep habits brought on by the coronavirus pandemic.

CPAP (continuous positive airway pressure): A therapy for patients with sleep apnea.

FED UP: An acronym I created to describe the toll the COVID-19 pandemic was having on us and our sleep: Financial stress, Emotional stress, Distance from others, Unpredictability, and Personal and professional stressors.

fragmentation: Frequent sleep disruptions in the middle of the night; "broken sleep."

GABA (gamma-aminobutyric acid): A chemical messenger that inhibits all of our wake-promoting centers and promotes sleep.

ghrelin: A hormone that makes you feel hungry.

homeostatic sleep drive: A natural process where your desire for sleep ramps up when you're awake and decreases while you sleep.

melatonin: A sleep hormone that signals our biological night and prepares us for sleep.

narcolepsy: A chronic sleep disorder marked by extreme daytime sleepiness; sufferers experience "sleep attacks" at inopportune times and may experience cataplexy (sudden loss of muscle tone with strong emotions such as laughter).

nocturia: Bathroom breaks at night (a.k.a. being a "loo hopper").

orthosomnia: An obsession with perfect sleep that's so extreme the person worries about sleep tracker data so much that they lose sleep.

ouch potato: Your snoring is so bad, you find yourself elbowed by your bed partner and end up sleeping on the couch.

parasomnias: Unusual events during sleep. Examples include sleepwalking, sleep terrors, sleep talking, sleep paralysis, sleep-related eating disorders, nightmares, and REM behavior disorder.

polysomnogram: A sleep study that gathers data from your brain and body during sleep.

primordial prevention: Having a plan *before* you have a health problem. In terms of sleep, it means following a plan and practicing better sleep habits now, even though there are no risk factors or signs of a disorder or problem. Primordial prevention is the ideal scenario in which all of us invest in better sleep every single night. It means filling up with good behaviors now so the bad ones have no space to grow.

REM: Rapid eye movement during sleep.

revenge bedtime procrastination: When people willingly put off their sleep to do something else even though they know they'll feel terrible in the morning.

sleep apnea: A sleep disorder in which snoring events, along with intermittent breathing pauses, occur repeatedly during sleep night after night.

Sleep Vigilante (alter ego of Dr. Abhinav Singh): A gentle warrior trained by trailblazers, this sleep mask–wearing defender of the night vanquishes sleep's villains with his potent cocktail of science, levity, and killer takeaways.

Sleep Vigilanteism: An enlightened, folksy, and sometimes thought-provoking observation about the universe of sleep from the Sleep Vigilante himself.

tandemic: An epidemic happening alongside (in tandem with) or caused by a pandemic. *Example:* More sleep problems were caused by the coronavirus pandemic.

ZQ: Your sleep quotient; the quality and health of your sleep.

Notes

Chapter 1: Sleep

1 "Edison's Electric Light," *New York Times*, September 5, 1882.

2 "Q & Abe Episode 1," President Lincoln's Cottage, August 1, 2019, https://www.lincolncottage.org/q-and-abe-episode-1/.

3 See James Maas, *Power Sleep* (New York: William Morrow Paperbacks, 1998).

4 E. Mignot, "Why We Sleep: The Temporal Organization of Recovery," *PLoS Biology* 6, no. 4 (2008): e106, https://doi.org/10.1371/journal.pbio.0060106.

5 A. Rechtschaffen, B. M. Bergmann, C. A. Everson, C. A. Kushida, and M. A. Gilliland, "Sleep Deprivation in the Rat: X. Integration and Discussion of the Findings," *Sleep* 12, no. 1 (February 1989): 68–87, PMID: 2648533.

6 I. Tobler and B. Schwierin, "Behavioural Sleep in the Giraffe (Giraffa camelopardalis) in a Zoological Garden," *Journal of Sleep Research* 5, no. 1 (March 1996): 21–32, https://onlinelibrary.wiley.com/doi/abs/10.1046/j.1365-2869.1996.00010.x.

7 E. Aserinsky and N. Kleitman, "Regularly Occurring Periods of Eye Motility, and Concomitant Phenomena, during Sleep," *Science* 118, no. 3062 (September 4, 1953): 273–74, https://www.science.org/doi/10.1126/science.118.3062.273.

8 Max Chafkin, "Yahoo!'s Marissa Mayer on Selling a Company While Turning It Around," Bloomberg Businessweek, August 4,

2016, https://www.bloomberg.com/features/2016-marissa-mayer
-interview-issue/.

9 Olga Khazan, "Thomas Edison and the Cult of Sleep Deprivation,"
   Atlantic, May 14, 2014.

10 Joanie Faletto, "Leonardo Da Vinci and Nikola Tesla Allegedly
   Followed the Uberman Sleep Cycle," Discovery.com, August 1, 2019,
   https://www.discovery.com/science/Uberman-SleepCycle.

11 "Sleeping Habits of Seven Most Powerful People," *Economic Times*,
   February 11, 2017.

12 Nathaniel F. Watson et al., "The Past Is Prologue: The Future of Sleep
   Medicine," *Journal of Clinical Sleep Medicine* 13, no. 1 (January 15,
   2017): 127–35, https://jcsm.aasm.org/doi/10.5664/jcsm.6406.

Chapter 2: The Hidden Truths of Sleep Loss

1 Apoorva Mandavilli, "The World's Worst Industrial Disaster Is Still
   Unfolding," *Atlantic*, July 10, 2018, https://www.theatlantic.com/
   science/archive/2018/07/the-worlds-worst-industrial-disaster-is
   -still-unfolding/560726/.

2 *Encyclopedia Britannica*, s.v. "Bhopal disaster," November 30, 2021,
   accessed June 4, 2022, https://www.britannica.com/event/Bhopal
   -disaster.

3 Sarah Keating, "The Boy Who Stayed Awake for 11 Days," BBC Future,
   January 18, 2018, https://www.bbc.com/future/article/20180118-the
   -boy-who-stayed-awake-for-11-days.

4 V. Shahly et al., "The Associations of Insomnia with Costly
   Workplace Accidents and Errors: Results from the America Insomnia
   Survey," *Archives of General Psychiatry* 69, no. 10 (2012): 1054–63,
   https://doi.org/10.1001/archgenpsychiatry.2011.2188.

5 "Evaluation of Safety Sensitive Personnel for Moderate-to-Severe
   Obstructive Sleep Apnea," Department of Transportation, July 31,
   2017, https://s3.amazonaws.com/public-inspection.federalregister
   .gov/2017-16451.pdf.

6 C. A. Everson, C. J. Henchen, A. Szabo, and N. Hogg, "Cell Injury and
   Repair Resulting from Sleep Loss and Sleep Recovery in Laboratory
   Rats," *Sleep* 37, no. 12 (2014): 1929–40, https://doi.org/10.5665/sleep
   .4244.

7 D. Dawson and K. Reid, "Fatigue, Alcohol and Performance
   Impairment," *Nature* 388, no. 235 (1997), https://doi.org/10.1038/
   40775.

8 Terry Young et al., "Sleep Disordered Breathing and Mortality: Eighteen-Year Follow-Up of the Wisconsin Sleep Cohort," *Sleep* 31, no. 8 (2008): 1071–78.

9 Hope Hodge Seck, "Captain Warned That Crew Wasn't Ready before Sub Ran Aground, Investigation Shows," Military.com, March 1, 2020, https://www.military.com/daily-news/2020/03/01/captain-warned-crew-wasnt-ready-sub-ran-aground-investigation-shows.html.

Chapter 3: The Sleep-Success Connection

1 Andrew M. Watson, "Sleep and Athletic Performance," *Current Sports Medicine Reports* 16, no. 6 (2017): 413–18, https://doi.org/10.1249/JSR.0000000000000418.

2 C. D. Mah, K. E. Mah, E. J. Kezirian, and W. C. Dement, "The Effects of Sleep Extension on the Athletic Performance of Collegiate Basketball Players," *Sleep* 34, no. 7 (2011): 943–50, https://doi.org/10.5665/SLEEP.1132.

3 American Academy of Sleep Medicine, "NFL, NBA, and NHL Teams Have a Disadvantage When Traveling West: Evening Games Show Greatest Disadvantage for Teams Traveling Westward," ScienceDaily, June 14, 2016, http://www.sciencedaily.com/releases/2016/06/160614133619.htm.

4 See Michael H. Smolensky and Lynne Lamberg, *The Body Clock Guide to Better Health* (New York: Henry Holt, 2000).

Chapter 4: The Best Kind of "Brainwashing"

1 Barbara Selby, "NASA Helps Pilots Combat Fatigue during Long Flights," NASA.gov press release, October 24, 1994, https://www.nasa.gov/home/hqnews/1994/94-177.txt.

2 A. R. Mendelsohn and J. W. Larrick, "Sleep Facilitates Clearance of Metabolites from the Brain: Glymphatic Function in Aging and Neurodegenerative Diseases," *Rejuvenation Research* 16, no. 6 (December 2013): 518–23, https://doi.org/10.1089/rej.2013.1530.

3 Ehsan Shokri-Kojori et al., "β-Amyloid Accumulation in the Human Brain after One Night of Sleep Deprivation," *Proceedings of the National Academy of Sciences* 115, no. 17 (April 24, 2018): 4483–88, https://www.pnas.org/doi/full/10.1073/pnas.1721694115.

4 S. Sabia et al., "Association of Sleep Duration in Middle and Old Age with Incidence of Dementia," *Nature Communications* 12, no. 2289 (April 20, 2021), https://doi.org/10.1038/s41467-021-22354-2.

5 Denise J. Cai et al., "REM, Not Incubation, Improves Creativity by Priming Associative Networks," *Proceedings of the National Academy of Sciences* 106, no. 25 (2009): 10130–34, https://www.pnas.org/doi/full/10.1073/pnas.0900271106.

6 E. B. Leary et al., "Association of Rapid Eye Movement Sleep with Mortality in Middle-Aged and Older Adults," *JAMA Neurology* 77, no. 10 (October 1, 2020): 1241–51, https://doi.org/10.1001/jamaneurol.2020.2108; erratum in *JAMA Neurology* 77, no. 10 (October 1, 2020): 1322, PMID: 32628261.

7 Ronald B. Postuma et al., "Parkinson Risk in Idiopathic REM Sleep Behavior Disorder: Preparing for Neuroprotective Trials," *Neurology* 84, no. 11 (2015): 1104–13, https://doi.org/10.1212/WNL.0000000000001364.

Chapter 5: 50 Ways Sleep Makes You Happy

1 Judith E. Carroll et al., "Partial Sleep Deprivation Activates the DNA Damage Response (DDR) and the Senescence-Associated Secretory Phenotype (SASP) in Aged Adult Humans," *Brain, Behavior, and Immunity* 51 (2016): 223–29, https://doi.org/10.1016/j.bbi.2015.08.024.

2 Judith E. Carroll et al., "Postpartum Sleep Loss and Accelerated Epigenetic Aging," *Sleep Health* 7, no. 3 (2021): 362–67, https://doi.org/10.1016/j.sleh.2021.02.002.

3 Adam J. Krause et al., "The Pain of Sleep Loss: A Brain Characterization in Humans," *Journal of Neuroscience* 39, no. 12 (March 20, 2019): 2291–2300, https://doi.org/10.1523/JNEUROSCI.2408-18.2018.

4 B. Sivertsen, T. Lallukka, K. J. Petrie, Ó. A. Steingrímsdóttir, A. Stubhaug, and C. S. Nielsen, "Sleep and Pain Sensitivity in Adults," *Pain* 156, no. 8 (August 2015): 1433–39, https://doi.org/10.1097/j.pain.0000000000000131.

5 Buse Keskindag and Meryem Karaaziz, "The Association between Pain and Sleep in Fibromyalgia," *Saudi Medical Journal* 38, no. 5 (2017): 465–75, https://doi.org/10.15537/smj.2017.5.17864.

6 Emily Charlotte Stanyer et al., "Subjective Sleep Quality and Sleep Architecture in Patients with Migraine: A Meta-analysis," *Neurology*

97, no. 16 (October 2021): e1620–e1631, https://doi.org/10.1212/WNL.0000000000012701.

7   Esther Donga et al., "A Single Night of Partial Sleep Deprivation Induces Insulin Resistance in Multiple Metabolic Pathways in Healthy Subjects," *Journal of Clinical Endocrinology & Metabolism* 95, no. 6 (June 1, 2010): 2963–68, https://doi.org/10.1210/jc.2009-2430.

8   Mounir Chennaoui et al., "How Does Sleep Help Recovery from Exercise-Induced Muscle Injuries?," *Journal of Science and Medicine in Sport* 24, no. 10 (2021): 982–87, https://doi.org/10.1016/j.jsams.2021.05.007.

9   I. Daghlas et al., "Sleep Duration and Myocardial Infarction," *Journal of the American College of Cardiology* 74, no. 10 (September 10, 2019): 1304–14, https://doi.org/10.1016/j.jacc.2019.07.022.

10 F. H. Kuniyoshi et al., "Day-Night Variation of Acute Myocardial Infarction in Obstructive Sleep Apnea," *Journal of the American College of Cardiology* 52, no. 5 (July 29, 2008): 343–46, https://doi.org/10.1016/j.jacc.2008.04.027.

11 E. Tasali, K. Wroblewski, E. Kahn, J. Kilkus, and D. A. Schoeller, "Effect of Sleep Extension on Objectively Assessed Energy Intake among Adults with Overweight in Real-Life Settings: A Randomized Clinical Trial," *JAMA Internal Medicine* 182, no. 4 (2022): 365–74, https://doi.org/10.1001/jamainternmed.2021.8098.

12 Christopher B. Cooper et al., "Sleep Deprivation and Obesity in Adults: A Brief Narrative Review," *BMJ Open Sport & Exercise Medicine* 4, no. 1 (October 4, 2018): e000392, https://doi.org/10.1136/bmjsem-2018-000392.

13 Faith S. Luyster et al., "Associations of Sleep Duration with Patient-Reported Outcomes and Health Care Use in US Adults with Asthma," *Annals of Allergy, Asthma & Immunology* 125, no. 3 (September 1, 2020): 319–24.

14 C. D. Mah, K. E. Mah, E. J. Kezirian, and W. C. Dement, "The Effects of Sleep Extension on the Athletic Performance of Collegiate Basketball Players," *Sleep* 34, no. 7 (2011): 943–50, https://doi.org/10.5665/SLEEP.1132.

15 T. Akerstedt, P. Fredlund, M. Gillberg, and B. Jansson, "A Prospective Study of Fatal Occupational Accidents—Relationship to Sleeping Difficulties and Occupational Factors," *Journal of Sleep Research* 11, no. 1 (March 2002): 69–71, https://onlinelibrary.wiley.com/doi/abs/10.1046/j.1365-2869.2002.00287.x.

16 Stoyan Dimitrov et al., "Gα$_s$-Coupled Receptor Signaling and Sleep Regulate Integrin Activation of Human Antigen-Specific T Cells," *Journal of Experimental Medicine* 216, no. 3 (March 4, 2019): 517–26.

17 A. A. Prather et al., "Temporal Links between Self-Reported Sleep and Antibody Responses to the Influenza Vaccine," *International Journal of Behavioral Medicine* 28 (2021): 151–58, https://doi.org/10 .1007/s12529-020-09879-4.

18 Sarah Gehlert et al., "Shift Work and Breast Cancer," *International Journal of Environmental Research and Public Health* 17, no. 24 (December 20, 2020): 9544, https://doi.org/10.3390/ijerph17249544.

19 B. K. J. Tan et al., "Association of Obstructive Sleep Apnea and Nocturnal Hypoxemia with All-Cancer Incidence and Mortality: A Systematic Review and Meta-analysis," *Journal of Clinical Sleep Medicine*, November 11, 2021, https://jcsm.aasm.org/doi/10.5664/ jcsm.9772, Epub ahead of print.

20 R. J. Reiter, "The Pineal Gland and Melatonin in Relation to Aging: A Summary of the Theories and of the Data," *Experimental Gerontology* 30, nos. 3–4 (May–August 1995): 199–212, https://doi.org/10.1016/ 0531-5565(94)00045-5; Thomas C. R. Vijayalaxmi Jr., R. J. Reiter, and T. S. Herman, "Melatonin: From Basic Research to Cancer Treatment Clinics," *Journal of Clinical Oncology* 20, no. 10 (May 15, 2002): 2575–601, https://doi.org/10.1200/JCO.2002.11.004.

21 Eti Ben Simon et al., "Losing Neutrality: The Neural Basis of Impaired Emotional Control without Sleep," *Journal of Neuroscience* 35, no. 38 (September 23, 2015): 13194–205, https://doi.org/10.1523/ JNEUROSCI.1314-15.2015.

22 G. G. Werner, M. Schabus, J. Blechert, and F. H. Wilhelm, "Differential Effects of REM Sleep on Emotional Processing: Initial Evidence for Increased Short-Term Emotional Responses and Reduced Long-Term Intrusive Memories," *Behavioral Sleep Medicine* 19, no. 1 (January–February 2021): 83–98, https://doi.org/10.1080/ 15402002.2020.1713134, Epub January 23, 2020.

23 Rosalba Hernandez et al., "The Association of Optimism with Sleep Duration and Quality: Findings from the Coronary Artery Risk and Development in Young Adults (CARDIA) Study," *Behavioral Medicine* 1 (2019), https://doi.org/10.1080/08964289.2019.1575179.

24 Peter L. Franzen and Daniel J. Buysse, "Sleep Disturbances and Depression: Risk Relationships for Subsequent Depression and Therapeutic Implications," *Dialogues in Clinical Neuroscience* 10, no. 4 (2008): 473–81, https://doi.org/10.31887/DCNS.2008.10.4/plfranzen.

25 E. Ben Simon, A. Rossi, A. G. Harvey, and M. P. Walker, "Overanxious and Underslept," *Nature Human Behaviour* 4, no. 1 (January 2020): 100–110, https://doi.org/10.1038/s41562-019-0754-8, Epub November 4, 2019; erratum in *Nature Human Behaviour* 4, no. 12 (December 2020): 1321, https://doi.org/10.1038/s41562-019-0754-8.

26 Danielle Pacheco, "Memory and Sleep," SleepFoundation.org, November 13, 2020, updated April 22, 2022, https://www.sleepfoundation.org/how-sleep-works/memory-and-sleep.

27 T. Åkerstedt et al., "Work and Sleep—a Prospective Study of Psychosocial Work Factors, Physical Work Factors, and Work Scheduling," *Sleep* 38, no. 7 (July 1, 2015): 1129–36, https://doi.org/10.5665/sleep.4828.

28 Matthew Gibson and Jeffrey Shrader, "Time Use and Productivity: The Wage Returns to Sleep," Department of Economics Working Papers 2015–17, Department of Economics, Williams College, 2015.

29 "Percentage of Adults Who Average ≤6 Hours of Sleep, by Family Income Group and Metropolitan Status of Residence," National Health Interview Survey, United States, April 3, 2015, https://www.cdc.gov/mmwr/preview/mmwrhtml/mm6412a10.htm.

30 Amy C. Reynolds et al., "Sickness Absenteeism Is Associated with Sleep Problems Independent of Sleep Disorders: Results of the 2016 Sleep Health Foundation National Survey," *Sleep Health* 3, no. 5 (2017): 357–61, https://doi.org/10.1016/j.sleh.2017.06.003.

31 Tina Sundelin et al., "Negative Effects of Restricted Sleep on Facial Appearance and Social Appeal," *Royal Society Open Science* 4 (2017): 160918160918.

32 E. Ben Simon and M. P. Walker, "Sleep Loss Causes Social Withdrawal and Loneliness," *Nature Communications* 9, no. 3146 (2018), https://doi.org/10.1038/s41467-018-05377-0.

33 Gary Wittert, "The Relationship between Sleep Disorders and Testosterone in Men," *Asian Journal of Andrology* 16, no. 2 (2014): 262–65, https://doi.org/10.4103/1008-682X.122586; R. Leproult and E. Van Cauter, "Effect of 1 Week of Sleep Restriction on Testosterone Levels in Young Healthy Men," *JAMA: Journal of the American Medical Association* 305, no. 21 (2011): 2173, https://doi.org/10.1001/jama.2011.710.

34 J. J. Pilcher et al., "Interactions between Sleep Habits and Self-Control," *Frontiers in Human Neuroscience* 9 (2015): 284, https://doi.org/10.3389/fnhum.2015.00284.

35 P. Huyett and N. Bhattacharyya, "Incremental Health Care Utilization and Expenditures for Sleep Disorders in the United States," *Journal of Clinical Sleep Medicine*, published online May 4, 2021, https://jcsm.aasm.org/doi/10.5664/jcsm.9392.

36 S. Sabia et al., "Association of Sleep Duration in Middle and Old Age with Incidence of Dementia," *Nature Communications* 12, no. 2289 (April 20, 2021), https://doi.org/10.1038/s41467-021-22354-2.

37 Terry Young et al., "Sleep Disordered Breathing and Mortality: Eighteen-Year Follow-Up of the Wisconsin Sleep Cohort," *Sleep* 31, no. 8 (2008): 1071–78.

Chapter 6: The ABCs of Zzzs

1 Lourdes M. DelRosso et al., "Consensus Diagnostic Criteria for a Newly Defined Pediatric Sleep Disorder: Restless Sleep Disorder (RSD)," *Sleep Medicine* 75 (2020): 335–40.

Chapter 7: Aging, and Sleeping, Gracefully

1 "2020 Profile of Older Americans," Administration for Community Living, U.S. Department of Health and Human Services, May 2021, https://acl.gov/sites/default/files/Aging%20and%20Disability%20in%20America/2020ProfileOlderAmericans.Final_.pdf.

2 Y. Naruse et al., "Concomitant Obstructive Sleep Apnea Increases the Recurrence of Atrial Fibrillation following Radiofrequency Catheter Ablation of Atrial Fibrillation: Clinical Impact of Continuous Positive Airway Pressure Therapy," *Heart Rhythm* 10, no. 3 (March 2013): 331–37, https://doi.org/10.1016/j.hrthm.2012.11.015, Epub November 23, 2012.

Chapter 8: While You Were Sleeping . . . during the Pandemic

1 J. Wouk et al., "Viral Infections and Their Relationship to Neurological Disorders," *Archives of Virology* 166, no. 3 (March 2021): 733–53, https://doi.org/10.1007/s00705-021-04959-6, Epub January 27, 2021.

2   K. M. Abel et al., "Association of SARS-CoV-2 Infection with
    Psychological Distress, Psychotropic Prescribing, Fatigue, and Sleep
    Problems among UK Primary Care Patients," *JAMA Network Open* 4,
    no. 11 (2021): e2134803, https://doi.org/10.1001/jamanetworkopen
    .2021.34803.

3   Matthew B. Maas et al., "Obstructive Sleep Apnea and Risk of
    COVID-19 Infection, Hospitalization and Respiratory Failure," *Sleep &
    Breathing = Schlaf & Atmung* 25, no. 2 (2021): 1155–57, https://doi.org/
    10.1007/s11325-020-02203-0.

4   L. Besedovsky, T. Lange, and M. Haack, "The Sleep-Immune
    Crosstalk in Health and Disease," *Physiological Reviews* 99, no. 3
    (July 1, 2019): 1325–80, https://doi.org/10.1152/physrev.00010
    .2018.

5   A. A. Prather, D. Janicki-Deverts, M. H. Hall, and S. Cohen,
    "Behaviorally Assessed Sleep and Susceptibility to the Common
    Cold," *Sleep* 38, no. 9 (September 1, 2015): 1353–59, https://doi.org/10
    .5665/sleep.4968.

Chapter 9: Fall in Love with Sleep Again

1   Kelly Glazer Baron et al., "Orthosomnia: Are Some Patients Taking
    the Quantified Self Too Far?," *Journal of Clinical Sleep Medicine* 13,
    no. 2 (February 15, 2017): 351–54, https://jcsm.aasm.org/doi/10
    .5664/jcsm.6472.

2   Hallie Levine, "Having Trouble Staying Asleep? 5 Strategies to
    Help You Fix Frequent Nighttime Awakenings," *Consumer Reports*,
    September 5, 2019, https://www.consumerreports.org/insomnia/
    having-trouble-staying-asleep-a9680912006/.

3   "New Year's Resolution: Don't Let COVID-somnia Drag You
    Down," AASM, December 28, 2021, https://aasm.org/new-years
    -resolution-dont-let-covid-somnia-drag-you-down/; "AASM Sleep
    Prioritization Survey: COVID-somnia," AASM, April 2021, https://
    j2vjt3dnbra3ps7ll1clb4q2-wpengine.netdna-ssl.com/wp-content/
    uploads/2021/04/sleep-prioritization-survey-2021-covid-somnia
    .pdf.

4   H. K. Khattak, F. Hayat, S. V. Pamboukian, H. S. Hahn, B. P. Schwartz,
    and P. K. Stein, "Obstructive Sleep Apnea in Heart Failure: Review
    of Prevalence, Treatment with Continuous Positive Airway Pressure,
    and Prognosis," *Texas Heart Institute Journal* 45, no. 3 (2018): 151–61,
    https://doi.org/10.14503/THIJ-15-5678.

Chapter 10: The Easy Sleep Reset

1 A. A. Borbély, S. Daan, A. Wirz-Justice, and T. Deboer, "The Two-Process Model of Sleep Regulation: A Reappraisal," *Journal of Sleep Research* 25, no. 2 (April 2016): 131–43, https://onlinelibrary.wiley.com/doi/10.1111/jsr.12371, Epub January 14, 2016.

Chapter 11: Cash in Your 13.5 Million

1 "Why Americans Can't Sleep," *Consumer Reports*, January 14, 2016.

Acknowledgments

Abhinav Singh's Acknowledgments

I would like to thank Vidhya, the most beautiful person that I end each day with and start each day beside. She makes me a better person every day. Thank you also to Zoe, our fierce, free-spirited 10-year-old who reminds me every day how irrelevant I am compared to her.

To my family: Thank you to my mom and dad and sister for always believing in and supporting me, and for tolerating all my eccentric idiosyncrasies. Thank you to Kumkum Aunty, who taught me to always stay positive no matter what.

I would like to say thank you to and honor the memory of Dr. Sharon Merritt, who first believed in me when I was new to the United States (just 14 days in this country). I wrote about her in the introduction; she interviewed me and hired me as an assistant for her sleep research. Dr. Merritt was the very first person to open the doors of the sleep research world to me, and it forever changed the course of my life.

I would like to acknowledge Dr. Bill Buffie, who hired me here fresh out of training and wrote this book's foreword, and Dr. Manfred Mueller, for all his support and mentorship—in addition to all my physician colleagues, including Dr. Steven Samuels, who trusted me with their patients. A special high-five to Dan Pankiewicz for helping us run the best sleep center ever.

Thank you to my agent, Greg Johnson, for believing in our project, and to our publisher, Humanix Books, who gave us this chance. Thank you to Roy Hibbert for sharing your journey to better sleep in this book and also to the entire Pacers organization.

To Charlotte Jensen, my gifted coauthor, without whom this dream project would have remained a dream: Her expert skill and linguistic genius helped me extract my vision and distill my experience into this enjoyable book, which will hopefully help spread the magic of sleep.

My background in sleep health would not be the same without the impacts of certain people along the way. I would like to thank Dr. Phyllis Zee, my mentor and an inspiring figure who gave me the opportunity by accepting me into her sleep fellowship program. Thank you for teaching me how to balance work, learning, and caring for patients, along with the importance of continuing to excel and learn every single day. It's impressive to watch her balance her global, thought-leading stature with running a busy department focusing on world-class research and filled with students, all with a smile and with authority.

My appreciation also goes to Dr. Rama Gourineni and Dr. Lisa Wolfe at Northwestern, as well as Dr. Joel Spear, my residency program director. He modeled how to be a good clinician and to think about always putting patients first. Because of him, I think, "Always do your best for the patient."

To Fred Meyer, who taught me "America" my first years here: He was like a fatherly figure to me at the research center, and he helped me assimilate here. I was this kid from Bombay (now Mumbai); there was so much I didn't know, and he helped me feel at ease being in a new and unfamiliar country. He taught me all the things that can't be taught from a book: how life works in America, the culture, the meanings of different phrases.

And to all my patients and their families, who put their faith and trust in me: You are the reason why I show up to work every day.

Charlotte Jensen's Acknowledgments

"Maybe we should write a book." It's amazing to think back to the very first time we said those words, when *Sleep to Heal* was just a tiny spark of an idea. But actually creating a book is an inspiring, challenging, rewarding process that never could have happened without the contributions and positive impacts of so many.

First to my son, who (innocently) deepened my understanding of sleep deprivation in the earliest months of his life: I'm so happy it was you keeping me company as I rocked your precious, extraordinary self under the stars in the wee hours. Thank you for inspiring me every single day and for continuing to teach me so much as you grow up.

To my coauthor, Abhinav Singh: This book literally could not exist without you, along with your brilliance, generosity, dedication, friendship, and contributions to the field of sleep health. Thank you for letting me share this incredible journey with you, for bringing joy to the process . . . and for helping me heal my own sleep along the way!

To Greg Johnson, who believed in our idea from the very first moment he read our proposal: Thank you for expertly shepherding this book for two debut authors still new to the process. Thank you also to Keith Pfeffer and the team at Humanix Books for your enthusiastic support and for making our dream of publishing a book a reality.

A very special thank you to Roy Hibbert: I'm so grateful you shared your very relatable story with our readers. I loved talking sleep, basketball, parenting, and even *Real Housewives* with you! Dr. Bill Buffie: Thank you for penning this book's foreword.

I'd also like to thank those wielding red pens, who helped me refine my craft along the way: from my high school English teachers; to my J-school college professors; to my first boss/editor, Diane Filipowski Stumpf; to Rieva Lesonsky and the talented team of editors (and now lifelong friends) formerly of *Entrepreneur* magazine.

Thank you to Mom and Dad for the bountiful bookshelves that surrounded me in childhood. And to my family: Maureen Lowe (for always checking in on me and celebrating my wins), Che Prasad (for fueling me with fancy dinners, sea shanties, and belly laughs), Kathleen Prasad (for believing in my writing), Susan Willis (for your love and encouragement), and Tom Brewster (for your wisdom).

Writing can feel lonely at times, and so to my dear friends Jenni Love (who paved the way by publishing her first book),

Diane Clark, Cynthia Merchant, Erica Perija, and Michi Duchon: Your good vibes, wine dates, encouraging texts, and FaceTimes made all the difference. Maria Geise: I credit your endless supply of gourmet Italian chocolates with magically preventing writer's block! To Shaun Chin, an exceptional listener and friend: You *always* held this unwavering belief that I would publish a book someday. (Wow, you were right!) Amanda Z., I owe so much gratitude to you for helping me find my way a few years back, when my dreams felt unreachable.

And finally, big hugs to my cat, Paddington, the best sleeper I know and my daily writing companion, who sprawled across my lap or keyboard for hours (usually purring) while this book slowly spun to life.

Index

About the Authors

Dr. Abhinav Singh is a physician with board certifications in sleep medicine and internal medicine. With a master's in public health and a keen interest in preventive medicine and promoting health, he firmly believes that better sleep equals better health. With a life mission of improving the world's sleep—one person, one night at a time—he is passionate about patients who have been diagnosed with sleep disorders and committed to making sure that they receive the best treatment plan, succeed with therapy, and regain restful sleep.

After receiving his medical degree, Dr. Singh completed his residency in internal medicine through the University of Illinois in Chicago at St. Joseph Hospital, followed by a fellowship in sleep medicine at Northwestern University. Currently, Dr. Singh serves as medical director at the Indiana Sleep Center, accredited by the American Academy of Sleep Medicine. He is also a clinical assistant professor at Marian University College of Osteopathic Medicine, where he developed and teaches a sleep medicine rotation to medical students. He is a fellow of the American Academy of Sleep Medicine and has received a Top Doctor award in sleep medicine for the last four years.

Dr. Singh is a peer reviewer for the *Journal of Clinical Sleep Medicine and Sleep Health* (a journal of the National Sleep Foundation). Dr. Singh regularly speaks at local, national, and global conferences and is a part of clinical trials relating to his specialty. He consults as a sleep physician for the NBA team the Indiana Pacers, serves on the medical review panel of SleepFoundation.org, and has been widely quoted in the media, including the *Washington Post*, the *Wall Street Journal*, *Martha Stewart Living*, HuffPost, CNET, *Glamour*, *Self*, *Prevention*, and other popular consumer lifestyle websites. Dr. Singh lives with his family in the greater Indianapolis metro area.

Charlotte Jensen is a writer and editor specializing in health, business, and tech topics. She previously spent more than a decade as senior writer, articles editor, and executive editor for *Entrepreneur* magazine, where she took a leading role in shaping editorial content and direction for the award-winning publication. Currently a copy editor for RH, her work has been featured in HuffPost and a variety of small-business websites. Jensen has a BA in journalism from California State University, Long Beach, and lives in beautiful Marin County, California, with her son and tabby Persian cat.